DATE DUE

12-1-05		
1-31-06		
3-15-07		
7-31-07		

Demco No. 62-0549

THIN *for* LIFE

Daybook

THIN *for* LIFE

Daybook

A Journal *of* Personal Progress—
Inspiration & Keys to Success
from People Who Have Lost Weight
& Kept It Off

Anne M. Fletcher, M.S., R.D.

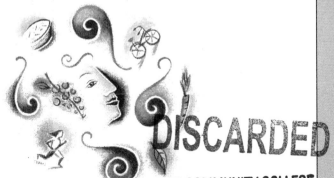

HOUGHTON MIFFLIN COMPANY

BOSTON   NEW YORK

1998

ISBN 1-57630-039-0

Printed in the United States of America
BP 10 9 8 7 6 5

Designed by Susan McClellan

Author's Note

As with all diets and weight-loss programs, you should obtain your physician's permission and seek his or her supervision before and while following the advice in the *Thin for Life Daybook*. This is particularly important if you have a medical problem, such as diabetes, high blood pressure or heart disease. A registered dietitian's counsel is advised as well. If you have psychological distress in your life, such as serious depression or high stress, you should see a psychologist or psychiatrist before following the *Thin for Life Daybook*'s recommendations. The author and publisher disclaim any liability arising directly or indirectly from the use of the *Thin for Life Daybook*.

All masters in the *Thin for Life Daybook* have given their permission to share information about their weight and eating habits. Some of their names have been changed to protect privacy and anonymity. Sometimes the masters' remarks were edited slightly for clarity.

Introduction

Learning from the Masters
of Weight Control

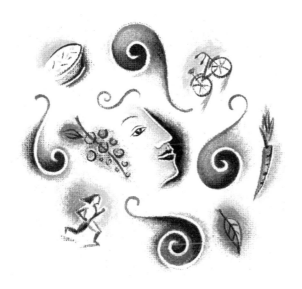

"Don't pay attention to the odds.
If you think you can't lose weight, you won't.
You have to ignore people who say you can't do it.
I had a terrible weight problem. It wasn't easy;
I'm not a superwoman. But I did it."

—Ann F. (220 pounds, 11 years)*

Wʜᴀᴛ ᴅɪᴅ Aɴɴ F. ᴅᴏ? She lost 220 pounds. Better still, she's kept it off for more than 11 years. Despite what you hear to the contrary, there are many, many people who, like Ann, have lost weight permanently. I know because I've devoted years to finding them and studying what it is that they do to be successful. I've personally located hundreds of individuals who have lost at least 20 pounds and kept their weight off for 3 or more years. I call these people "masters of weight control." And masters they are: Of the more than 200 successful people I've surveyed, their average weight loss is 64 pounds, and the average length of time they've been masters is more than 10 years. *Who better to tell you how to slim down than the very people who have done it?* I share their secrets and keys to success in my books *Thin for Life* and *Eating Thin for Life.*

Now, it's one thing to say you're going to lose weight; it's another thing altogether to put into effect a day-by-day plan to actually get rid of unwanted pounds. The real trick, if you want to *keep* the weight off, is to develop weight-control strategies you can use on a daily basis and to build on them for a lifetime. We're talking about changing *for good*—a proposition that can seem overwhelming if you don't take it one step at a time. Based on the advice from the masters, the *Thin for Life Daybook* takes you through a step-by-step process of permanently changing your eating habits, your weight and, ultimately, your life.

---

*When two numbers are given after a person's name, the first refers to the number of pounds the person has lost and the second to the length of time that person has been a master of weight control.

Note that the *Daybook* is not a diet and does not include a diet, although you may choose to use one, with your doctor's permission. You can start the *Daybook* at any point, according to your needs and what interests you at the time.

For each of 52 weeks, the *Daybook* provides the following:

❖ **"Weekly Wisdom"**—a message or lesson to inspire and guide you. The Weekly Wisdoms are based on the common threads that have led the masters of weight control to success. You'll learn how to change your mind-set and habits concerning food and weight, one step at a time.

❖ **"Weekly Forecast"**—space for you to set weekly goals, anticipate obstacles and make an exercise plan.

❖ **Meals from the Masters**—ideas for satisfying low-fat breakfasts, lunches, suppers and snacks, based on the masters' favorites, from my book *Eating Thin for Life.*

❖ **"Weekly Diary"**—two pages for keeping track of what you eat and how you exercise each day, as well as to record your successes and plan ahead.

As you work through the *Daybook*, note that it's a *combination* of strategies that works for long-term weight control. Don't feel compelled to do everything at once—the *Daybook* helps you take it week by week, day by day. In the words of Julie R., who's been master of a 53-pound weight loss for 13 years, *"Master one change before you make another."*

Setting Goals You Can Reach

*"When you focus on having to lose 100 pounds,
you think, 'What the hell; two more cookies isn't going
to make a difference.' But you can do it if you learn to set
your goals just for today or just for this meal. Then you
don't have to think about having to lose 100 pounds."*

—*Lois M. (72 pounds, 4 years)*

L OIS IS TALKING ABOUT ESTABLISHING REALISTIC GOALS that don't set you up for failure. Unfortunately, however, dieters often set vague goals like, "I'll be thin by summer" or unrealistic goals such as, "I'll never eat chocolate again." Sure, you might be successful for a while, but vague and unrealistic goals usually cannot be sustained.

For these reasons, an important part of the *Daybook* is setting one or two "Goals for this week." Here are some guidelines for planning your goals:

1. **Base your goals on where you are now,** not on some unrealistic standard. For instance, if you've been eating sweets three times a day, it's more realistic to cut back to once a day or three times a week than to replace all the sweets in your diet with fruit. Similarly, if you want to change your long-standing habit of skipping breakfast, it may help to start out having a small bowl of cereal rather than planning a hot meal that includes all of the food groups.

2. **Don't set "never" or "always" goals.** They're usually too perfectionist and cannot be maintained in the long run. So, instead of swearing off chocolate forever, make your goal to eat it only in controlled situations, as in a restaurant where portions are predetermined or when you can split a dessert with a friend.

3. Set goals that are specific and action-oriented. Rather than resolve, "I am going to eat healthier" or "I'm going to get in shape," try, "I'm going to switch from sugar-coated to a tasty high-fiber cereal with fruit" or "I'm going to walk on my lunch hour three times this week." It helps, too, to focus on short-term goals. Rather than saying, "I'll be thin by summer," think about what you can do "just for now" to start moving yourself in that direction, such as having fruit and some pretzels at coffee break rather than a Danish.

4. Be ready to change your goals. If you keep failing to meet a goal, perhaps you need to scale it down. If having dessert only three times a week doesn't work for you, try having something each night, but watch the portion size and try to find reduced-fat alternatives. Also, you may choose to work on some of your goals for more than one week—until you find you've got them down pat.

5. Give yourself praise for any and all accomplishments, be they large or small. Since dieters so often focus on their shortcomings, it's important to go back through your day and mentally note all the things you "did right." They may be relatively big steps, such as packing your lunch instead of giving in to the temptations of a cafeteria at work. Or you may list small accomplishments, such as using skim milk instead of 2-percent on your cereal. The *Daybook* gives you a place to do this *each day* in the diary sections marked Exercise/Accomplishments. (Your accomplishments need not be food- or exercise-related—if you feel good about cleaning out a cupboard or finishing your income taxes, record that as well so you learn to be more positive.)

Learning to set realistic goals and focus on small successes will spur you on: One success breeds another.

Anticipating Obstacles

"Once I accept the responsibility for a problem,
it eases. I say to myself, 'What can I do about that?'
Then I work on a solution so it doesn't happen again.
That way, I'm looking the problem right in the eye
instead of getting out of my worries by eating."
—*Tom F. (65 pounds, 20 years)*

D AY-TO-DAY CHALLENGES CAN SABOTAGE your efforts at weight loss. The obstacles can be out of your control, such as the death or illness of a loved one. But there are also many small challenges each week that you *can* anticipate and prepare for. Thus, each week in the Weekly Forecast there is a place to record "Anticipated Obstacles" and "Possible Solutions."

The obstacle to your weight-loss efforts could be a dinner party on Friday night, a business trip, a particularly stressful day in the week ahead or that plateful of doughnuts sitting next to the coffee pot at work each day. After you itemize the potential obstacles for the week to come, list at least one possible solution or way of getting around each obstacle to avoid overeating.

When you are not successful, don't berate yourself: Come up with an idea for handling the problem next time. When you *are* successful, be sure to note your triumphs. At the end of each week, record in the section "What Really Helped" those steps that were particularly beneficial in managing your weight and your eating. At the end of the year, you'll have a rich library of techniques to turn back to whenever you need a shot in the arm.

Coming Up with an Exercise Plan

*"Regular exercise helped me burn calories and reduce
stress that triggers overeating. I was able to gradually replace
my food 'addiction' with physical activity. Exercise has
helped me feel better, get control over my life
and feel good about myself."*

—*Dorothy C. (28 pounds, 11 years)*

YOU PROBABLY DON'T NEED DOROTHY to tell you that exercise helps tremendously with weight control. Indeed, when I asked the masters how they were finally successful at *losing* weight, their most consistent response was "exercise." When I asked them to list the three most important things they do to *maintain* weight loss, three out of four of them included exercise. And when I asked the masters to tell me what they do if they *gain* some weight, the most common answer was "Exercise more."

But most masters are not exercise fanatics. Few do so every day, and not many are marathon runners; walking is their number-one form of exercise. Experts suggest that what's most important about exercise is consistency and enjoyment and less so the amount or type of activity. The truth is that any exercise is better than none, and even modest amounts can bring about significant health and psychological benefits. The idea is to come up with a plan you can live with so that exercise becomes part of your life—just like brushing your teeth or putting on your seat belt. I think it's fair to say that most people who become hooked on exercise can't imagine their lives without it.

So how do you get hooked and stay hooked? As with finding the right way to lose weight, the word from the masters is, *You have to find what's right for you.*

In finding the form of exercise that's right for you on a regular basis, ask yourself the following questions:

❖ Is the form of exercise enjoyable or at least not unenjoyable? If you hate doing it, you'll likely give it up quickly.

❖ Is there a financial cost involved, and can you afford it on an ongoing basis? If you can't swing a fancy health club, you may want to consider a YMCA, YWCA or community center.

❖ Is it convenient? The greater the effort to get somewhere or work it into your schedule, the less likely you'll stick with it.

❖ Do you prefer privacy and solitary workouts or are you more of a group exerciser or someone who would be more motivated with an exercise buddy?

ONCE YOU SETTLE ON THE TYPE OF EXERCISE you'd like to do, the next step is to set realistic goals, just as with your eating habits. If you've been a couch potato for decades, don't think you're going to start out running—or even walking—a mile a day. (Interestingly, the drop-out rate for vigorous exercise programs has been reported to be much higher than that for moderate-intensity programs.)

Your short-term goal should be to start doing something—anything—to get yourself moving. Ernie L., master of a 45-pound weight loss, started "small" by running one minute a day and slowly worked upward. If you decide to walk for 15 minutes every other day and find you can do more, you'll feel very accomplished. But if you decide to work out every day for an hour and end up doing only two days for 20 minutes, you may feel like a failure. After you have accomplished your minimum goal for several weeks, then you can add on another day of exercise and/or another 5 to 10 minutes to your routine.

One thing *not* to do is to leave your exercising to chance—or say you'll do it only if you feel like it. It's important to think ahead and have some sort of game plan. So, for each week on the Weekly Forecast page, map out your exercise plan. Look at your daily schedule to see where exercise would best fit in—for instance, first thing in the morning, during your lunch hour or right after work.

Also, it is probably wise to vary your exercise—most masters engage in two or more forms such as walking and cycling. Variety helps to prevent tedium.

Don't feel compelled to exercise every day, and realize that your goals should be flexible. If, for instance, you have a bad headache or an unexpected late meeting at work, you may choose to take the day off from your 30-minute walk and make up for it another day, or you could cut back to 15 minutes, figuring any exercise is better than none. As you go through the week, record what you *actually* did.

Before starting any kind of exercise regime, get your physician's permission, particularly if you are overweight or have/had any medical problems, including heart disease or heart problems of any sort, chest pain, high blood pressure, diabetes or orthopedic or musculoskeletal problems. You should also get medical approval for exercise if you have not engaged in vigorous activity for a long time or if you are a 40-plus-year-old man or a woman aged 50 or above.

Don't Go It Alone

*"Just as any professional athlete needs a coach, sometimes you
need someone with an objective eye outside yourself."*
—*Steve S. (210 pounds, 13 years)*

THE MORE I LOOKED AT THE MASTERS' RESPONSES to my
question, "When you were finally successful, how did you
lose the weight?" the more I was struck by the diversity of their responses. About half of them were "program people," having lost
weight with help—most commonly from commercial weight-loss
programs or self-help groups. The other half were what I call "self-
styled" masters; they lost weight on their own, typically by following low-fat, low-calorie, sensible food plans and increasing exercise.
There were also lots of individual techniques that helped the masters lose weight, such as eating smaller portions, counting calories,
keeping diet diaries and changing the timing of their meals. (Week
11 helps you decide whether you're a program person or a self-
styler.)

No matter how you do it, losing weight—and keeping it off—
can be a lonely proposition. *But you don't have to go it alone.* Many
masters turn to others for support, some on a regular basis, others
as needed. In fact, weight-control experts have determined that
support from family, friends and maintenance support groups is
associated with long-term success at weight control.

Support can come in the form of individual counseling from a
registered dietitian or psychologist, a weight-loss program, or a
caring spouse, friend or relative. Not only can a support system give
you assurance that you're not alone, it can provide advice and new
ideas. It can also help with getting your problems in perspective and
heighten your accountability to yourself—say, by encouraging you
to "weigh in" at each meeting. Not everyone needs intense, long-
term support. Some masters needed more in the beginning—when

their weight loss was new—while others need reinforcement for a much longer period of time, perhaps forever. Many masters now go it alone, some seeking support when they feel themselves slipping.

Cindy F., for instance, regained a fair amount of weight after having her first baby but mustered up the courage to return to Weight Watchers, weighing in at 210 pounds. She told me, "I decided, 'I'm not going back up to 285 pounds.' In the past, I was a spokesperson for Weight Watchers, so it was hard to go back. But I found the support I needed and met others in the same situation."

What's important is that you view your recognition of the need for support as a sign of strength, not weakness.

Keeping a Food Diary

THE PURPOSE OF KEEPING A FOOD DIARY is to keep track of every calorie-containing item that you eat. For each day of the diary, be sure to record *everything* you consume, including snacks and beverages. (There is no need to write down items that are calorie-free or close to it, such as black coffee or diet beverages.) A food diary has several benefits:

❖ It can help you identify areas for improvement in your eating habits. For instance, if you feel you should be losing weight but seem to be at a standstill, go back and look at your diary to see where the extra calories may be coming from.

❖ It can help you recognize patterns in your eating habits that may be getting in the way of weight loss. For example, after a week or so of keeping records, you may see that you are consuming too many high-calorie items right when you come home from work. That may tell you to have a diet soda at that time of day or to plan ahead for a low-calorie snack.

❖ It makes you accountable for your own behavior. When you write down everything, you are forced to be aware of what you're eating. It can also prevent problem eating: You may find yourself thinking, "I don't want to eat that handful of peanuts because I'll have to write it down."

It is also important to note that the vast majority of masters told me that they plan ahead for meals and snacks. You don't have to map out every single detail about your future food plans, but at least give some thought to what you'll be eating in the day ahead so your food choices are not left to chance.

Goal(s) for this week: ① Get up 10 minutes earlier on weekdays so there's time for breakfast.
② Have 5 fruits & vegetables a day.

Anticipated Obstacles

- To New York tues.- 2 meals in restaurants

- Dinner party fri.- late dinner.

Possible Solutions

- Order same types of foods I'd have at home. Take fruit for snacks.

- Have light snack @ 6:00 PM

Exercise Plan

Monday: Walk 20 min. w/Sue & Holly at work / lunch hour

Tuesday: Day off

Wednesday: Same as Monday

Thursday: Same

Friday: Same

Saturday: Bicycle 40 min. after breakfast (stationary bike if rainy)

Sunday: Day off

Try This for Breakfast

❖ **Breakfast Shake:** 6 ounces strawberry yogurt (nonfat, sweetened with aspartame), 1 medium banana, 1 tablespoon wheat germ, ⅓ cup skim milk, ¼ cup orange juice. Combine all ingredients in a blender until smooth.

Calories: 270   Fat: 1.5 grams   (Katie G.)

Weekly Diary

Monday

What I Ate:

MORNING
2 cups coffee w/2T
½ + ½ each
½ c raisin bran w/
2 sliced strawberries
+ ½ c skim milk
10:00 – 1 banana

AFTERNOON
Bagel w/ 1oz. low-fat
cream cheese
15 grapes
6 baby carrots
2 hard candies
4:00 – tea w/skim milk
6 animal crackers

EVENING
3"x3" cheese omelette
1 c. green beans
1 roll w/ 1 pat margarine
2 gum drops
10:00 – 1 c. vanilla frozen
yogurt

Exercise / Accomplishments: Had breakfast/had 4 fruits + veg /walked 20 min.

Tuesday

What I Ate:

MORNING
2 cups coffee w/2T
½ + ½
¾ c. mini shredded wheat
½ sliced banana
¾ c. skim milk
10:00 – 1 plain donut

AFTERNOON
Turkey club:
3 slices wheat bread
3 slices tomato
1 slice provolone
3 slices smoked turkey
Dijon mustard
3:00 – large apple

EVENING
6 oz. filet mignon
1 med. baked potato w/
low-fat Ranch dressing
large tossed salad w/
low-fat dressing
6 stalks asparagus
key lime pie – shared.

Exercise / Accomplishments:
Fruit for snack/shared dessert /had breakfast/careful in restaurant.

Wednesday

What I Ate:

MORNING
1 English muffin
w/2 Tsp. jam
¼ cantaloupe
4 cups coffee w/
2T ½ + ½

AFTERNOON
1½ c. vegetable soup
1 oz. low-fat cheese
5 melba rounds
1 large orange
4:00 – 1 pear / 10 low-fat
tortilla chips

EVENING
3"x4" piece lasagne
1 slice Italian bread
3 stalks broccoli
2 c. spinach salad w/3T
low-fat Ital. dressing
1 c. skim milk
10:00 – 1" slice watermelon

Exercise / Accomplishments:
Breakfast /5 a day! /Walked 20 min.

Thursday

What I Ate:

MORNING
½ c. raisin bran w/
½ c. skim milk
1 slice wheat toast w/
apple butter
2 cups coffee
w/ 2T ½ + ½

AFTERNOON
1 blueberry yogurt (6oz.)
20 pretzel sticks
1 large apple
4:00 – tea w/skim
milk
1 plain biscotti cookie

EVENING POTLUCK
(went a little crazy...)
a little of this & that–
casseroles, jellomold,
coleslaw, veggies, dip,
apple crisp –
oh well!

Exercise / Accomplishments:
Didn't keep eating after Potluck/walked 15 min./packed lunch.

Weekly Diary

Friday

What I Ate:

MORNING

1 fat-free peach
  yogurt (6oz.)
½ grapefruit
1 slice wheat toast w/
  1 tsp. diet margarine
2 cups coffee w/2T
  ½ + ½

AFTERNOON

½ tuna sub
1 med. nectarine
1 c. skim milk
_____
10 small pretzels
6 oz. orange juice

EVENING

Veggies + dip
4 oz. broiled salmon
1 c. rice
1 c. steamed spinach
  w/ bacon bits
½ c. chocolate mousse

Exercise / Accomplishments: Took steps instead of elevator 5 times.

Saturday

What I Ate:

MORNING

1 whole wheat bagel
1 oz. Neufchatel
2 cups coffee w/
  2T ½ + ½

AFTERNOON

2 slices w. bread w/
  1 T mayo (low-fat)
3 slices turkey breast
½ med. tomato
1 med. apple
1 choc. chip cookie

EVENING (Restaurant)

6 oz. glass red wine
2 slices garlic bread
2 manicotti in tomato
  sauce
2 c. Caesar salad
¾ c. raspberry sorbet

Exercise / Accomplishments:
½ hour bicycling / had low-fat dessert in restaurant.

Sunday

What I Ate:

MORNING

2 poached eggs
½ English muffin w/
  lt. butter
⅛ cantaloupe
2 cups coffee w/
  2T ½ + ½

AFTERNOON

1 c. leftover
  spaghetti w/ tomato sauce
1 meatball
1 med. nectarine
5 Jordan almonds
later- 15 tortilla chips
¼ c. salsa; 6 oz. w. wine

EVENING

4 oz. grilled flank steak
½ twice-baked potato
4 broccoli spears
1½ c. Romaine lettuce
  w/ 2 T low-fat Ranch
Snack- 1 c. mint-chip ice
  cream

Exercise / Accomplishments: Had 5 fruits + vegetables.

What Really Helped This Week:

- Anticipating food choices for the next day.

- Having breakfast (less tempted mid-morning).

- Talking to Diane when stressed out.

- Having a healthy snack before the party.

I

Psyching Yourself Up

Getting the Right Mind-Set
to Lose Weight

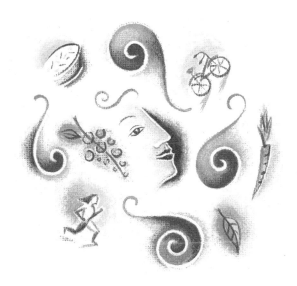

Believe that you can become thin for life.

*"I was desperate after 30 years of diets.
When I saw my first Weight Watchers leader—
thin and healthy—I was inspired! I saw people maintaining
50 to 100-pound weight losses. I could do, and I did ."*

—*Doris M. (71 pounds, 24 years)*

THE MESSAGE FROM THE MASTERS IS, "If you think you can, you will." Over and over, they describe moving from a state of hopelessness to one of self-control and power. They began to believe in their own ability to take charge, and they stopped seeing themselves as passive victims of their weight.

So how can you start to believe in yourself? It helps to observe role models—people who have struggled to master situations that you fear or see as difficult.

Identify one person in your everyday life who is taking positive steps to be healthy and control his or her weight. That person does not have to be a "master" or even someone who is thin—just someone who is trying. It could be an acquaintance you regularly see mall-walking, a neighbor who frequently jogs past your house or someone you notice making healthful food choices at work. Ask the person how he or she stays motivated. Tell yourself, "If this person can do it, I can do it, too."

_____

_____

_____

_____

Goal(s) for this week: _____

_____

_____

Anticipated Obstacles   **Possible Solutions**

_____   _____

_____   _____

_____   _____

Exercise Plan

Monday: _____

Tuesday: _____

Wednesday: _____

Thursday: _____

Friday: _____

Saturday: _____

Sunday: _____

Try This for Breakfast

❖ ⅓ cup uncooked oatmeal prepared with 8 ounces skim milk. Top with ½ tablespoon strawberry or raspberry jam. ❖ 6 ounces freshly squeezed orange juice.

Calories: 297   **Fat: 2.5 grams**   (Dean M.)

WEEK

1

What I Ate: ———————— Monday ————————

MORNING   AFTERNOON   EVENING

Exercise / Accomplishments:

What I Ate: ———————— Tuesday ————————

MORNING   AFTERNOON   EVENING

Exercise / Accomplishments:

What I Ate: ———————— Wednesday ————————

MORNING   AFTERNOON   EVENING

Exercise / Accomplishments:

What I Ate: ———————— Thursday ————————

MORNING   AFTERNOON   EVENING

Exercise / Accomplishments:

What I Ate: —————— **Friday** ——————

MORNING   AFTERNOON   EVENING

Exercise / Accomplishments:

What I Ate: —————— **Saturday** ——————

MORNING   AFTERNOON   EVENING

Exercise / Accomplishments:

What I Ate: —————— **Sunday** ——————

MORNING   AFTERNOON   EVENING

Exercise / Accomplishments:

—————— **What Really Helped This Week:** ——————

Free yourself from the myths about weight control.

*"When I had thoughts like 'You failed in the past,'
I tried to push them out of my mind and replace them with
positive images. I wanted to be the person that I knew
was in there waiting to come out."*

—**Kay D. (102 pounds, 3 years)**

I T'S TIME TO STOP LISTENING TO THE FAILURE TALK—about how almost no one succeeds at losing weight and keeping it off. The masters shatter myth after myth about weight control:

Myth #1: If you've been overweight since childhood, you'll never succeed. *(Seven out of ten masters had been heavy since their youth.)*

Myth #2: There's no hope for yo-yo dieters. *(Most masters tried to lose weight at least five times before finally succeeding.)*

Myth #3: You have to eat like a bird to keep weight off. *(Many masters eat several meals a day, often with snacks and treats in between.)*

This week, free yourself from the myths by doing the following:

❖ Each time you feel discouraged, remind yourself of at least one positive image or goal you have set for yourself.

❖ Focus on what you *can* have rather than on deprivation. List five (or more) special low-fat treats you will have this week, such as ripe berries, frozen yogurt, warm bagels or fresh sea scallops.

_____

_____

_____

_____

_____

Goal(s) for this week: _____

_____

_____

Anticipated Obstacles   **Possible Solutions**

_____   _____

_____   _____

_____   _____

Exercise Plan

Monday: _____

Tuesday: _____

Wednesday: _____

Thursday: _____

Friday: _____

Saturday: _____

Sunday: _____

Try This for Lunch

❖ **Soft-Shelled Chicken Taco:** 1 flour tortilla (8 inches), 2 ounces cooked chicken breast (in strips), ¼ cup salsa, ⅓ cup shredded lettuce, 1 ounce shredded reduced-fat cheddar cheese, 2 tablespoons nonfat sour cream ❖ ½ cup red grapes.

Calories: 400   **Fat: 10 grams**   (Don C.)

What I Ate: ———————— Monday ————————

MORNING   AFTERNOON   EVENING

Exercise / Accomplishments:

What I Ate: ———————— Tuesday ————————

MORNING   AFTERNOON   EVENING

Exercise / Accomplishments:

What I Ate: ———————— Wednesday ————————

MORNING   AFTERNOON   EVENING

Exercise / Accomplishments:

What I Ate: ———————— Thursday ————————

MORNING   AFTERNOON   EVENING

Exercise / Accomplishments:

What I Ate: ———————— **Friday** ————————————

MORNING   AFTERNOON   EVENING

Exercise / Accomplishments:

What I Ate: ———————— **Saturday** ————————

MORNING   AFTERNOON   EVENING

Exercise / Accomplishments:

What I Ate: ———————— **Sunday** ————————

MORNING   AFTERNOON   EVENING

Exercise / Accomplishments:

———————— **What Really Helped This Week:** ————————

Realize that if you're fat, it may not be your fault—but you can still do something about it.

"This time I felt in control. It was not an act of fate that I was heavy, not bad luck. I knew it was up to me to change."
—**Donna C., on her final weight-loss attempt (88 pounds, 5 years)**

I F YOU COME FROM A LINE OF HEAVY PEOPLE or you've been overweight for a long time, you can throw up your hands *or* you can do something about it. The masters are living proof that weight destiny need not be controlled by your genes or by the fact that you're a "slow burner" of food.

It's true that experts are finding weight problems to be, in part, caused by "bad" genes and faulty metabolism. One person may need 2,300 calories a day to maintain weight, but another of the same weight, height, age and activity level may require just 1,500 calories. Not everyone is meant to be skinny.

Note, however, that it's a *tendency* to become overweight that's inherited. In many cases heaviness results from the *combination* of a genetic predisposition, unhealthy eating habits and inadequate physical activity. It's easy to fall into the trap of using the genetic argument as an excuse.

What are some excuses you make about your weight?

_____

_____

This week, when you find yourself falling into the "excuse mentality," take one small step. For instance, walk around the block, wait 20 minutes before you indulge a craving or call a friend instead of eating.

Goal(s) for this week: _____

_____

_____

Anticipated Obstacles   **Possible Solutions**

_____   _____

_____   _____

_____   _____

Exercise Plan

Monday: _____

Tuesday: _____

Wednesday: _____

Thursday: _____

Friday: _____

Saturday: _____

Sunday: _____

Try This for Supper

❖ 4 ounces grilled teriyaki chicken breast ❖ 1½ cups broccoli, with nutmeg and lemon juice ❖ 6 small red-skin potatoes, roasted in 2 teaspoons olive oil and crushed garlic ❖ 1 cup coleslaw: 1 cup shredded cabbage, 1 teaspoon sugar, 2 tablespoons nonfat mayonnaise and 2 teaspoons Dijon mustard.

Calories: 486   **Fat: 14.5 grams**   (Jim V.)

Monday

What I Ate:

MORNING　　　　　AFTERNOON　　　　　EVENING

Exercise / Accomplishments:

Tuesday

What I Ate:

MORNING　　　　　AFTERNOON　　　　　EVENING

Exercise / Accomplishments:

Wednesday

What I Ate:

MORNING　　　　　AFTERNOON　　　　　EVENING

Exercise / Accomplishments:

Thursday

What I Ate:

MORNING　　　　　AFTERNOON　　　　　EVENING

Exercise / Accomplishments:

Friday

What I Ate:

MORNING   AFTERNOON   EVENING

Exercise / Accomplishments:

Saturday

What I Ate:

MORNING   AFTERNOON   EVENING

Exercise / Accomplishments:

Sunday

What I Ate:

MORNING   AFTERNOON   EVENING

Exercise / Accomplishments:

What Really Helped This Week:

Set a comfortable weight goal.

*"I wanted to be 123, but my recommended weight is higher.
Also, I don't want to deprive myself and be obsessive about
exercise in order to lose. I'm a size 10 and that's OK."*

—*Jennifer P. (56 pounds, 15 years)*

IF YOU'RE LIKE MOST PEOPLE WHO DECIDE TO SLIM DOWN, the first thing you do is set a weight goal, such as "I'm going to get down to 125." But many masters have accepted themselves at a heavier weight than they once deemed ideal—their "comfortable" weight.

**In setting your comfortable weight goal,
let the following guide you:**

❖ As an adult, what's the lowest weight you've ever been able to maintain for at least a year? _____ (It may be difficult to comfortably maintain a lower weight.)

❖ At what weight can you say to yourself, "I look quite good given where I've been?" _____

❖ Think of acquaintances who look "normal" to you, not like models. Find out if they mind your asking what they weigh.

❖ At what weight can you live with the required changes in eating and/or exercise? _____

If you feel constantly hungry or if you have to exercise more than is realistic, your comfortable weight is higher.*

* This exercise is based on guidelines by weight-control experts Drs. Kelly Brownell, Judith Rodin and Thomas Wadden.

Goal(s) for this week: _____

_____

_____

Anticipated Obstacles	Possible Solutions
_____	_____
_____	_____
_____	_____

Exercise Plan

Monday: _____

Tuesday: _____

Wednesday: _____

Thursday: _____

Friday: _____

Saturday: _____

Sunday: _____

Try This for Dessert

❖ 1½-ounce slice low-fat pound cake, topped with ⅓ cup sliced
fresh strawberries and ¼ cup fat-free strawberry frozen yogurt.

Calories: 190   Fat: 2.5 grams   (Thalia A.)

What I Ate: ———————— **Monday** ————————

MORNING   AFTERNOON   EVENING

Exercise / Accomplishments:

What I Ate: ———————— **Tuesday** ————————

MORNING   AFTERNOON   EVENING

Exercise / Accomplishments:

What I Ate: ———————— **Wednesday** ————————

MORNING   AFTERNOON   EVENING

Exercise / Accomplishments:

What I Ate: ———————— **Thursday** ————————

MORNING   AFTERNOON   EVENING

Exercise / Accomplishments:

What I Ate: ——————— Friday ———————

MORNING   AFTERNOON   EVENING

Exercise / Accomplishments:

What I Ate: ——————— Saturday ———————

MORNING   AFTERNOON   EVENING

Exercise / Accomplishments:

What I Ate: ——————— Sunday ———————

MORNING   AFTERNOON   EVENING

Exercise / Accomplishments:

——————— What Really Helped This Week: ———————

Take responsibility for your weight.

"When I finally realized that I wasn't doing it for my parents but for me—that's when I felt successful."

—*Jim V. (235 pounds, 5 years)*

THE LAST TIME YOU LOST WEIGHT, were you really doing it for yourself—or for someone else? Taking responsibility seemed to be the critical starting point for many masters. They came to terms with the fact that they had to want to lose the weight primarily for themselves and that no one was going to do it for them.

**Here are some ideas that may help you
take responsibility for your weight:**

1. *Accept what you can't change.* There comes a time when you have to stop complaining, "Why me? It's not fair," and ask yourself, "What am I going to do about it?"

2. *Face the truth.* Before you can take responsibility, you first have to be honest with yourself. List one or two ways that you've been kidding yourself (for instance, "At least I'm not as fat as my sister" or "It's my husband's fault because he buys junk food").

_____

_____

3. *Do it for you.* Who are you losing the weight for?

_____

If your response isn't, first and foremost, "for me," then you may not be ready to lose weight. *The desire has to come from within.*

Weekly Forecast

Goal(s) for this week: _____

_____

_____

Anticipated Obstacles   **Possible Solutions**

_____   _____

_____   _____

_____   _____

Exercise Plan

Monday: _____

Tuesday: _____

Wednesday: _____

Thursday: _____

Friday: _____

Saturday: _____

Sunday: _____

Try This for Breakfast

❖ 1 poached egg sprinkled with 1 teaspoon bacon bits ❖ 1 slice
whole wheat toast with 1 tablespoon raspberry jam ❖ 6 ounces
grapefruit juice.

Calories: 294   **Fat: 7 grams**   (Joy C.)

Weekly Diary

What I Ate: ——————— Monday ———————

MORNING   AFTERNOON   EVENING

Exercise / Accomplishments:

What I Ate: ——————— Tuesday ———————

MORNING   AFTERNOON   EVENING

Exercise / Accomplishments:

What I Ate: ——————— Wednesday ———————

MORNING   AFTERNOON   EVENING

Exercise / Accomplishments:

What I Ate: ——————— Thursday ———————

MORNING   AFTERNOON   EVENING

Exercise / Accomplishments:

Friday

What I Ate:

MORNING   AFTERNOON   EVENING

Exercise / Accomplishments:

Saturday

What I Ate:

MORNING   AFTERNOON   EVENING

Exercise / Accomplishments:

Sunday

What I Ate:

MORNING   AFTERNOON   EVENING

Exercise / Accomplishments:

What Really Helped This Week:

Want to be thinner more than you want to eat the "wrong" foods.

"I feel better physically. My clothes fit better. Women find me attractive. I am healthier. I don't have to dread going out in public. Nothing tastes as good as being thin feels. What more motivation do I need?"

—*Ted H. (142 pounds, 6 years)*

T HE MASTERS HAVE REACHED THE POINT where the benefits of being thinner far overshadow the effort involved. It's worth it to them to make some sacrifices and changes to obtain what they get in return.

For some people, it helps to look within, asking these critical questions:

❖ How do I feel about myself at this weight, and how does that conflict with what I'd like to be and do?
❖ How would I feel if I lost weight?

Make a list of the "pros" of losing weight—what you'll get out of being thinner. Then make a list of "cons," or the drawbacks involved in losing weight.

PROS   CONS

_____   _____

_____   _____

_____   _____

_____   _____

You'll be ready to lose weight for good when the pros mean more to you than the cons.

Goal(s) for this week: _____

_____

_____

Anticipated Obstacles	Possible Solutions
_____	_____
_____	_____
_____	_____

Exercise Plan

Monday: _____

Tuesday: _____

Wednesday: _____

Thursday: _____

Friday: _____

Saturday: _____

Sunday: _____

Try This for Lunch

❖ **Chinese Chicken Salad:** Toss together 3 ounces cooked, cubed skinless chicken breast, 2 cups shredded cabbage, ½ red or green pepper (sliced), ¼ cup sliced green onions, 1 teaspoon sugar, 1 teaspoon sesame seeds, ½ tablespoon sesame oil. Season with salt or soy sauce, vinegar or lemon juice and pepper. Top with ¼ cup chow mein noodles ❖ ¾ cup pineapple chunks (fresh or in juice).

Calories: 386   Fat: 15.5 grams   (Judy F.)

What I Ate: ———————— Monday ————————

MORNING   AFTERNOON   EVENING

Exercise / Accomplishments:

What I Ate: ———————— Tuesday ————————

MORNING   AFTERNOON   EVENING

Exercise / Accomplishments:

What I Ate: ———————— Wednesday ————————

MORNING   AFTERNOON   EVENING

Exercise / Accomplishments:

What I Ate: ———————— Thursday ————————

MORNING   AFTERNOON   EVENING

Exercise / Accomplishments:

What I Ate: ———————— Friday ————————

MORNING   AFTERNOON   EVENING

Exercise / Accomplishments:

What I Ate: ———————— Saturday ————————

MORNING   AFTERNOON   EVENING

Exercise / Accomplishments:

What I Ate: ———————— Sunday ————————

MORNING   AFTERNOON   EVENING

Exercise / Accomplishments:

———————— What Really Helped This Week: ————————

Prepare yourself to lose weight.

"My weight is something I will have to struggle with all my life. But I've accepted it. And it definitely gets easier with time."

—*Cindy P. (80 pounds, 12 years)*

IN ORDER TO BE SUCCESSFUL, the masters first had to accept some things about themselves and the weight-maintenance process.

❖ *Accept that it's not easy, not always fair.* Losing weight and keeping it off may be one of the hardest things you ever do. It may help to remind yourself that many things you've wanted have taken some effort. List one or more difficult efforts that have paid off:

_____

_____

❖ *Realize that your motivation for weight control will wax and wane.* What are some steps you can take to keep yourself going? (For example, buy several outfits in your new size, take photos of yourself and post them next to old "heavy" ones, get out of the house at night.)

_____

_____

❖ *Get in touch with what your weight is doing for you.* Being heavy enables some people to put off making decisions or taking action. What are some things you've put off doing "until you lose weight"?

_____

_____

WEEK

7

Weekly Forecast

Goal(s) for this week: _____

_____

_____

Anticipated Obstacles   Possible Solutions

_____   _____

_____   _____

_____   _____

Exercise Plan

Monday: _____

Tuesday: _____

Wednesday: _____

Thursday: _____

Friday: _____

Saturday: _____

Sunday: _____

Try This for Supper

❖ 1 cup fresh strawberries ❖ 3 ounces roasted turkey breast (skinless)
❖ ½ cup scalloped potatoes (made with skim milk and reduced-
calorie margarine) ❖ ½ cup fresh green beans, steamed ❖ 1 medium
ear corn on the cob ❖ **Salad:** 1 cup romaine lettuce, ⅓ cup
cauliflower florets, 3 cherry tomatoes, ½ red pepper (sliced),
½ medium carrot (sliced), 3 tablespoons fat-free blue cheese dressing.

Calories: 499   **Fat: 5.5 grams**   (Rose B.)

What I Ate: ———————— Monday ————————

MORNING   AFTERNOON   EVENING

Exercise / Accomplishments:

What I Ate: ———————— Tuesday ————————

MORNING   AFTERNOON   EVENING

Exercise / Accomplishments:

What I Ate: ———————— Wednesday ————————

MORNING   AFTERNOON   EVENING

Exercise / Accomplishments:

What I Ate: ———————— Thursday ————————

MORNING   AFTERNOON   EVENING

Exercise / Accomplishments:

What I Ate: ——————— Friday ———————

MORNING   AFTERNOON   EVENING

Exercise / Accomplishments:

What I Ate: ——————— Saturday ———————

MORNING   AFTERNOON   EVENING

Exercise / Accomplishments:

What I Ate: ——————— Sunday ———————

MORNING   AFTERNOON   EVENING

Exercise / Accomplishments:

——————— What Really Helped This Week: ———————

Get ready for down the road.

"I've enjoyed the compliments—and disbelief—
regarding my weight loss and improved appearance.
My energy level is better. I'm more active, outgoing and self-assured.
I'm attractive to men. And most important, I like myself!"

—Donna C. (88 pounds, 5 years)

IT HELPS TO KNOW THE PLUSES AND MINUSES of what you may encounter when you're thinner.

❖ *Prepare for the "hardship" of being thin.* Some masters say they wish they'd known that there might be some negative changes after first losing weight. For instance, heavy friends and relatives sometimes try to sabotage your efforts. Members of the opposite sex may react to you in new ways. You may have trouble accepting your thin self.

List at least one "hardship" you may face after slimming down and come up with a possible way to handle it. (For instance, your husband may be jealous of other men.)

_____

_____

❖ *Look forward to what you'll gain.* The masters report far more favorable changes in their lives than negative ones.

What do you look forward to when you lose weight?

_____

_____

_____

Goal(s) for this week: _____

_____

_____

Anticipated Obstacles

Possible Solutions

_____ _____

_____ _____

_____ _____

Exercise Plan

Monday: _____

Tuesday: _____

Wednesday: _____

Thursday: _____

Friday: _____

Saturday: _____

Sunday: _____

Try This for Breakfast

❖ 1 blueberry bagel (2½ ounces) with 2 teaspoons nonfat cream cheese ❖ **Skinny Latte**: 8 ounces strong coffee with 8 ounces steamed skim milk.

Calories: 300   Fat: 2.5 grams   (Judy C.)

What I Ate: ———————— Monday ————————

MORNING   AFTERNOON   EVENING

Exercise / Accomplishments:

What I Ate: ———————— Tuesday ————————

MORNING   AFTERNOON   EVENING

Exercise / Accomplishments:

What I Ate: ———————— Wednesday ————————

MORNING   AFTERNOON   EVENING

Exercise / Accomplishments:

What I Ate: ———————— Thursday ————————

MORNING   AFTERNOON   EVENING

Exercise / Accomplishments:

Friday

What I Ate:

MORNING   AFTERNOON   EVENING

Exercise / Accomplishments:

Saturday

What I Ate:

MORNING   AFTERNOON   EVENING

Exercise / Accomplishments:

Sunday

What I Ate:

MORNING   AFTERNOON   EVENING

Exercise / Accomplishments:

What Really Helped This Week:

Make a lifelong commitment.

*"Most people think they can go back to their former eating habits,
which made them fat in the first place. You can't. You can allow a few
more treats and eat a few larger meals on special occasions,
but you must still watch it at other times."*

—*Shirley G. (85 pounds, 20 years)*

BE HONEST. When you've tried to lose weight in the past, were you secretly hoping you'd be able to eat whatever you wanted after you got down to your goal? The masters have accepted a permanent new way of living, thinking and eating.

It's easier to commit to lifestyle change if you are reasonably stable and happy.

Ask yourself the following questions:

❖ Is my financial situation stable? _____
❖ Is my job likely to stay the same for at least a year? _____
❖ Is my workload manageable and will it likely stay that way? _____
❖ Am I willing to find time to devote to weight control? _____
❖ Can I find a way to become more physically active? _____
❖ Am I willing to put up with some discomfort in my eating or exercise habits to accomplish my goal? _____
❖ Are my family members reasonably healthy? _____
❖ Are my relationships reasonably healthy? _____
❖ Do these people support my efforts to lose weight? _____
❖ Overall, am I happy right now? _____
❖ Can I accept that I will have to make an effort to lose weight? _____

In general, the more "yeses" you have, the closer you are to being ready to take charge of your weight once and for all.

Weekly Forecast

Goal(s) for this week: _____

_____

_____

Anticipated Obstacles　　**Possible Solutions**

_____　　_____

_____　　_____

_____　　_____

Exercise Plan

Monday: _____

Tuesday: _____

Wednesday: _____

Thursday: _____

Friday: _____

Saturday: _____

Sunday: _____

Try This for Lunch

❖ 1 medium baked potato, cut into chunks. Serve on a bed of 2 cups tossed salad topped with 3 tablespoons fat-free Catalina dressing. ❖ 6 ounces strawberry yogurt (nonfat, sweetened with aspartame) ❖ 1 medium orange.

Calories: 398　　　　Fat: 1 gram　　　　(Patsy B.)

Weekly Diary

What I Ate: —————————— Monday ——————————

MORNING   AFTERNOON   EVENING

Exercise / Accomplishments:

What I Ate: —————————— Tuesday ——————————

MORNING   AFTERNOON   EVENING

Exercise / Accomplishments:

What I Ate: —————————— Wednesday ——————————

MORNING   AFTERNOON   EVENING

Exercise / Accomplishments:

What I Ate: —————————— Thursday ——————————

MORNING   AFTERNOON   EVENING

Exercise / Accomplishments:

What I Ate: ———————— Friday ————————

MORNING   AFTERNOON   EVENING

Exercise / Accomplishments:

What I Ate: ———————— Saturday ————————

MORNING   AFTERNOON   EVENING

Exercise / Accomplishments:

What I Ate: ———————— Sunday ————————

MORNING   AFTERNOON   EVENING

Exercise / Accomplishments:

——————— What Really Helped This Week: ———————

Give yourself time.

*"Take it a day at a time. When I started, not only
was I overweight, but I had little confidence in myself.
So I decided to do it 5 pounds at a time. I didn't look at losing
75 to 80 pounds, because I figured that was going
to set me up for failure."*

—*Kay D. (102 pounds, 3 years)*

LIKE YOU, THE MASTERS DIDN'T GAIN WEIGHT OVERNIGHT, and they didn't lose it in a week or a month, either. The vast majority of masters took six or more months to reach their goal weights.

If you decide to go to a weight-loss program, the longer you stick with it, the more weight you'll likely lose and the greater the odds are that you'll keep it off. No matter how you tackle your weight problem, it's important to be patient, weathering those inevitable "plateaus."

To remind yourself of your ability to be patient, list below some other accomplishment(s) in life you feel proud of. (For example, finishing your college degree, figuring out how to build something from scratch or learning how to play the piano. Note, too, how long it took you to complete the task or to become proficient at the new skill.)

_____

_____

_____

_____

_____

Goal(s) for this week: _____

_____

_____

Anticipated Obstacles   **Possible Solutions**

_____   _____

_____   _____

_____   _____

Exercise Plan

Monday: _____

Tuesday: _____

Wednesday: _____

Thursday: _____

Friday: _____

Saturday: _____

Sunday: _____

Try This for Breakfast

❖ **Yogurt "Sundae":** Layer in a brandy snifter ¼ cup fresh blueberries, ½ peach (sliced), ¼ cup sliced strawberries, 4 ounces raspberry yogurt (nonfat, sweetened with aspartame). Repeat and top with 3 tablespoons reduced-fat granola.

Calories: 286   **Fat: 2 grams**   (Ann F.)

What I Ate: ———————— Monday ————————

MORNING   AFTERNOON   EVENING

Exercise / Accomplishments:

What I Ate: ———————— Tuesday ————————

MORNING   AFTERNOON   EVENING

Exercise / Accomplishments:

What I Ate: ———————— Wednesday ————————

MORNING   AFTERNOON   EVENING

Exercise / Accomplishments:

What I Ate: ———————— Thursday ————————

MORNING   AFTERNOON   EVENING

Exercise / Accomplishments:

What I Ate: ——————— Friday ———————

MORNING   AFTERNOON   EVENING

Exercise / Accomplishments:

What I Ate: ——————— Saturday ———————

MORNING   AFTERNOON   EVENING

Exercise / Accomplishments:

What I Ate: ——————— Sunday ———————

MORNING   AFTERNOON   EVENING

Exercise / Accomplishments:

——————— What Really Helped This Week: ———————

II

Getting It Off

Taking Charge of Your Weight

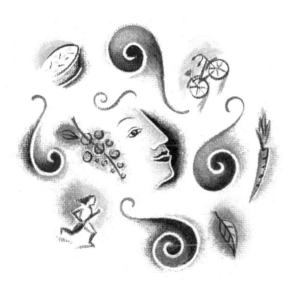

Learn from the past.

*"What works for one may not work for another.
If you hate fish, don't eat it just to lose weight."*

—*Sam E. (46 pounds, 12 years)*

WHEN YOU'RE READY TO ACTIVELY LOSE WEIGHT, what's the best way? No matter what you currently weigh or how many times you've lost and regained, you are more knowledgeable now than you were in the past. As Ernie L. puts it, "You get to be an expert because you had so many failures."

Reflect on your last several weight-loss attempts:

❖ What was the food plan or diet like? Was the calorie level too high or too low? What foods could you have? What foods couldn't you have?

❖ How did you feel—both physically and mentally?

❖ What sort of exercise plan did you follow? Was it realistic? How could you modify it?

❖ Did you adopt new activities that were helpful?

What worked	What didn't work
having occasional treats	strict dieting
eating three meals a day	skipping lunch
packing lunch the night before	eating soup five times a day
_____	_____
_____	_____
_____	_____

Think about your answers as you decide how to lose weight.

$$\textit{Weekly Forecast}$$

Goal(s) for this week: _____

_____

_____

Anticipated Obstacles	Possible Solutions
_____	_____
_____	_____
_____	_____

Exercise Plan

Monday: _____

Tuesday: _____

Wednesday: _____

Thursday: _____

Friday: _____

Saturday: _____

Sunday: _____

Try This for Lunch

❖ **Sandwich:** 1 ounce lean corned beef on 2 slices low-calorie wheat bread, with 3 large leaves leaf lettuce and Dijon mustard ❖ 6 fat-free potato chips ❖ 1 fat-free fig bar ❖ 1 cup chocolate milk (8 ounces skim milk with 2 tablespoons chocolate syrup).

Calories: 384   **Fat: 4.5 grams**   (Shirley C.)

What I Ate: —————— Monday ——————
MORNING   AFTERNOON   EVENING

Exercise / Accomplishments:

What I Ate: —————— Tuesday ——————
MORNING   AFTERNOON   EVENING

Exercise / Accomplishments:

What I Ate: —————— Wednesday ——————
MORNING   AFTERNOON   EVENING

Exercise / Accomplishments:

What I Ate: —————— Thursday ——————
MORNING   AFTERNOON   EVENING

Exercise / Accomplishments:

What I Ate: ———————— Friday ————————

MORNING   AFTERNOON   EVENING

Exercise / Accomplishments:

What I Ate: ———————— Saturday ————————

MORNING   AFTERNOON   EVENING

Exercise / Accomplishments:

What I Ate: ———————— Sunday ————————

MORNING   AFTERNOON   EVENING

Exercise / Accomplishments:

———————— What Really Helped This Week: ————————

When you're ready to lose weight, do it your way.

*"I am convinced that permanent weight loss is something
each individual must work out for himself. For me, it was a
combination of exercise, psychological and philosophical enlightenment
and healthy diet. You have to look at your eating style
and see what will work for you."*

—*Ernie L. (40 pounds, 17 years)*

THE MASTERS' MESSAGE—loud and clear—is that if you want to lose weight, you have to find what's best for you. You have to do it your way.

About half of the masters lost weight with the help of weight-loss programs and/or professionals. The other half did it on their own.

**If you agree with all or most of the following statements,
you're more likely to be a self-styler:**

—— I prefer to deal with things on my own.

—— I dislike group activities.

—— I've had it with weight-loss programs.

—— I can come up with my own food and exercise plan.

If you disagree, you'll want to shop around for a program that's right for you. Do some research, discussing the matter with your physician and/or a dietitian, or consult the Yellow Pages. Take into consideration the program's affordability and convenience.

Before choosing a program, ask yourself if it:

—— Supports setting a "comfortable" weight goal.

—— Emphasizes exercise, but in a realistic way for my lifestyle.

—— Has a food plan I can live with, at least for a while.

—— Has a comprehensive maintenance program.

Weekly Forecast

Goal(s) for this week: _____

_____

_____

Anticipated Obstacles   **Possible Solutions**

_____   _____

_____   _____

_____   _____

Exercise Plan

Monday: _____

Tuesday: _____

Wednesday: _____

Thursday: _____

Friday: _____

Saturday: _____

Sunday: _____

Try This for Supper

❖ 4-ounce grilled rib-eye steak (weight after trimming and cooking)
❖ 1 medium baked potato (4 ounces) with 1 tablespoon real sour
cream with chives ❖ ½ cup steamed peas ❖ ⅙ medium cantaloupe.

Calories: 498   **Fat: 17 grams**   (Jean B.)

What I Ate: ——————— Monday ————————

MORNING   AFTERNOON   EVENING

Exercise / Accomplishments:

What I Ate: ——————— Tuesday ————————

MORNING   AFTERNOON   EVENING

Exercise / Accomplishments:

What I Ate: ——————— Wednesday ————————

MORNING   AFTERNOON   EVENING

Exercise / Accomplishments:

What I Ate: ——————— Thursday ————————

MORNING   AFTERNOON   EVENING

Exercise / Accomplishments:

What I Ate: ——————— Friday ———————

MORNING   AFTERNOON   EVENING

Exercise / Accomplishments:

What I Ate: ——————— Saturday ———————

MORNING   AFTERNOON   EVENING

Exercise / Accomplishments:

What I Ate: ——————— Sunday ———————

MORNING   AFTERNOON   EVENING

Exercise / Accomplishments:

——————— What Really Helped This Week: ———————

To diet or not to diet? You decide.

*"In the past, my problem was that I focused on 'the diet'
and what I had to give up. I was either 'going on' or 'going off.'
Then I went to a class taught by a dietitian that emphasized
behavior modification, exercise and fat reduction."*

—**Donna C. (88 pounds, 5 years)**

IT ALMOST GOES WITHOUT SAYING that to lose weight, you have to eat less than you're currently eating. So do you go on a diet or do you follow a nondieting approach—simply cutting back and trying to eat more healthful foods?

Although a number of masters said that they did best without a diet, planned diets did work for many of them.

To figure out if you're a candidate for dieting, consider the following:

❖ Have I done well on diets in the past? _____

❖ Do I like guidance and structure? _____

❖ If I go on a formal diet, will it give me enough leeway to include foods that I really like? If not, am I prepared to make short-term sacrifices? _____

To decide if you want to go the nondieting route, ask yourself:

❖ Do I feel confident that I can come up with your own healthful eating plan? _____ (You may want to make an appointment with a registered dietitian at your hospital's outpatient department to get started.)

❖ If I want to lose weight quickly on a medically supervised program, can I afford the cost? _____ (If not, a less expensive group program that offers a calorie-restricted food plan may be for you.)

No one solution applies to all individuals.

Goal(s) for this week: _____

_____

_____

Anticipated Obstacles   Possible Solutions

_____   _____

_____   _____

_____   _____

Exercise Plan

Monday: _____

Tuesday: _____

Wednesday: _____

Thursday: _____

Friday: _____

Saturday: _____

Sunday: _____

Try This for Breakfast

❖ 1 slice whole wheat toast with 1 tablespoon reduced-fat peanut butter ❖ 8 ounces skim milk flavored with 1 teaspoon almond extract and 1 packet low-calorie sweetener.

Calories: 274   Fat: 7.5 grams   (Jennifer B.)

What I Ate: —————————— Monday ——————————

MORNING   AFTERNOON   EVENING

Exercise / Accomplishments:

What I Ate: —————————— Tuesday ——————————

MORNING   AFTERNOON   EVENING

Exercise / Accomplishments:

What I Ate: —————————— Wednesday ——————————

MORNING   AFTERNOON   EVENING

Exercise / Accomplishments:

What I Ate: —————————— Thursday ——————————

MORNING   AFTERNOON   EVENING

Exercise / Accomplishments:

What I Ate: ——————— Friday ———————

MORNING   AFTERNOON   EVENING

Exercise / Accomplishments:

What I Ate: ——————— Saturday ———————

MORNING   AFTERNOON   EVENING

Exercise / Accomplishments:

What I Ate: ——————— Sunday ———————

MORNING   AFTERNOON   EVENING

Exercise / Accomplishments:

——————— What Really Helped This Week: ———————

WEEK

14

Get rid of the excuses for not exercising.

*"When I stop exercising for a bit, my weight goes up.
When I increase my activity, I go back to normal. Remember:
There are 24 hours in a day, and you should be able
to find one for yourself."*

—*Jim V. (235 pounds, 5 years)*

DO YOU FIND YOURSELF MAKING EXCUSES to get out of exercise? The masters make exercise a regular, nonnegotiable part of their lives.

**Check which of the following excuses for exercise you use,
and come up with ways to challenge them:**

❖ "I don't have time." The masters stress that you have to make exercise a priority. _____ _____

❖ "I'm too tired." Actually, many people find that exercising gives them an energy boost. _____ _____

❖ "I'm too old." It's never too late to find some way to be more physically active. _____ _____

❖ "I'm too self-conscious." Shop around for an exercise class for heavier people. _____ _____

❖ "It's too hot/it's too cold." Find an indoor, temperature-controlled place, like a mall or YMCA, to work out.

_____ _____

❖ "My friends and family are not supportive." Try to get an unsupportive person to exercise with you.

_____ _____

This week, give yourself an excuse for exercising. Buy one new exercise-related product or article of clothing to psych yourself.

Goal(s) for this week: _____

_____

_____

Anticipated Obstacles   Possible Solutions

_____   _____

_____   _____

_____   _____

Exercise Plan

Monday: _____

Tuesday: _____

Wednesday: _____

Thursday: _____

Friday: _____

Saturday: _____

Sunday: _____

Try This for Lunch

❖ Cheese soufflé, made with 2 eggs and 2 ounces fat-free cheddar cheese ❖ 1 slice sourdough bread ❖ ¾ cup applesauce (no sugar added), sprinkled with cinnamon.

Calories: 378   Fat: 11 grams   (Jennie C.)

Monday

What I Ate: ————————————————

MORNING   AFTERNOON   EVENING

Exercise / Accomplishments:

Tuesday

What I Ate: ————————————————

MORNING   AFTERNOON   EVENING

Exercise / Accomplishments:

Wednesday

What I Ate: ————————————————

MORNING   AFTERNOON   EVENING

Exercise / Accomplishments:

Thursday

What I Ate: ————————————————

MORNING   AFTERNOON   EVENING

Exercise / Accomplishments:

What I Ate: ———————— Friday ————————

MORNING   AFTERNOON   EVENING

Exercise / Accomplishments:

What I Ate: ———————— Saturday ————————

MORNING   AFTERNOON   EVENING

Exercise / Accomplishments:

What I Ate: ———————— Sunday ————————

MORNING   AFTERNOON   EVENING

Exercise / Accomplishments:

———————— What Really Helped This Week: ————————

Make a lasting commitment to exercise.

*"One of the keys to sticking with exercise is to vary the routine.
It helps that I enjoy aerobics, but after 11 years, I do need to use
all kinds of 'tricks' to stay motivated: special music tapes, new classes,
gyms and machines, new clothing, running with my husband."*

—***Dorothy C. (28 pounds, 11 years)***

EXERCISE DOESN'T HAVE TO BE DRUDGERY—the masters find pleasurable ways to be active. As Ann B. states, "I found things to do that I enjoyed, so exercise wasn't a chore."

The masters also tend to vary their exercise: six out of ten of them do at least two different forms. They may walk one day, take a light aerobics class the next. Some make changes with the season, bicycling outdoors when the weather's nice and doing indoor aerobics in the wintertime.

Most masters give themselves days off—the majority do not exercise every day. Some of them play positive mind games, focusing on the payoff rather than the labor of exercise. For instance, when Kim W. was getting hooked on exercise, she fantasized about being a dancer. Don't make it a catastrophe when you fall short of your exercise goal. A day missed here and there doesn't even amount to a pound of weight gain. *Make a special effort this week to make your exercise more enjoyable, for instance, by listening to music or walking with a friend.*

**Write down what worked so you have ideas next time
you get into an exercise slump:**

_____

_____

_____

_____

Goal(s) for this week: _____

_____

_____

Anticipated Obstacles   **Possible Solutions**

_____   _____

_____   _____

_____   _____

Exercise Plan

Monday: _____

Tuesday: _____

Wednesday: _____

Thursday: _____

Friday: _____

Saturday: _____

Sunday: _____

Try This for Supper

❖ **Eggplant Parmesan:** 5 slices eggplant baked with ½ cup reduced-fat spaghetti sauce and 1 ounce shredded part-skim mozzarella cheese ❖ ½ cup cooked angel hair pasta ❖ **Salad:** 1½ cups iceberg lettuce, ¼ cup bean sprouts, ½ cucumber (sliced), ½ medium tomato (sliced), 2 tablespoons reduced-calorie Italian dressing ❖ 1-ounce breadstick ❖ ½ medium papaya.

Calories: 489   Fat: 8.5 grams   (Ann F.)

Weekly Diary

What I Ate: ———————— Monday ————————————

MORNING   AFTERNOON   EVENING

Exercise / Accomplishments:

What I Ate: ———————— Tuesday ————————————

MORNING   AFTERNOON   EVENING

Exercise / Accomplishments:

What I Ate: ———————— Wednesday ————————

MORNING   AFTERNOON   EVENING

Exercise / Accomplishments:

What I Ate: ———————— Thursday ————————————

MORNING   AFTERNOON   EVENING

Exercise / Accomplishments:

What I Ate: ———— **Friday** ————

MORNING   AFTERNOON   EVENING

Exercise / Accomplishments:

What I Ate: ———— **Saturday** ————

MORNING   AFTERNOON   EVENING

Exercise / Accomplishments:

What I Ate: ———— **Sunday** ————

MORNING   AFTERNOON   EVENING

Exercise / Accomplishments:

———— **What Really Helped This Week:** ————

Make your routine activities count.

*"When I go to a mall, I park my car far away from the entrance.
I always take the stairs at work."*

—Jim V. (235 pounds, 5 years)

DO YOU GO OUT OF YOUR WAY to find the nearest parking spot at the mall or supermarket? Do you take escalators instead of the steps beside them? Merely walking up and down two flights of stairs a day instead of using an elevator can shed 5 or 6 pounds each year!

**Check off the "little" activities below
that you could add to your daily routine:**

____ At work and/or at home, go out of your way to use a bathroom or get a drink of water on a different floor.

____Park your car at a far spot in a parking lot.

____Get off the bus or have the cab drop you off a block or two before your destination.

____Upon arrival at your place of work, take the stairs at least part of the way to your floor.

____Move your wastebasket to a place in your office that forces you to get up when something has to be discarded. (No shooting baskets!)

____In airports, don't use moving walkways.

____When you need to speak with someone, walk to the next room rather than raise your voice.

____Walk your dog.

____Sit in a rocking chair and rock as you watch TV.

____Hide the remote control.

Little activities add up.

Goal(s) for this week: _____

_____

_____

Anticipated Obstacles   **Possible Solutions**

_____   _____

_____   _____

_____   _____

Exercise Plan

Monday: _____

Tuesday: _____

Wednesday: _____

Thursday: _____

Friday: _____

Saturday: _____

Sunday: _____

Try This for a Snack

❖ Baked sweet potato (5 ounces), sliced and microwaved with
⅓ cup miniature marshmallows on top.

Calories: 196   **Fat: negligible**   (Dorothy C.)

What I Ate: —————— Monday ——————

MORNING   AFTERNOON   EVENING

Exercise / Accomplishments:

What I Ate: —————— Tuesday ——————

MORNING   AFTERNOON   EVENING

Exercise / Accomplishments:

What I Ate: —————— Wednesday ——————

MORNING   AFTERNOON   EVENING

Exercise / Accomplishments:

What I Ate: —————— Thursday ——————

MORNING   AFTERNOON   EVENING

Exercise / Accomplishments:

What I Ate: ———————— **Friday** ————————

MORNING   AFTERNOON   EVENING

Exercise / Accomplishments:

What I Ate: ———————— **Saturday** ————————

MORNING   AFTERNOON   EVENING

Exercise / Accomplishments:

What I Ate: ———————— **Sunday** ————————

MORNING   AFTERNOON   EVENING

Exercise / Accomplishments:

———————— **What Really Helped This Week:** ————————

If you want it, have it.

*"There is nothing I completely avoid.
I don't have as many cravings now that I eat a little of everything.
Depriving yourself totally is not the key."*

—*Shirley G. (85 pounds, 20 years)*

THE MASTERS HAVE BROKEN FREE from the deprivation syndrome—they've reached the point where they can eat "just one" without remorse, knowing they can have it again. When I asked them how they deal with cravings, their number-one response was, "*I have a little.*"

Some masters started having favorite foods while they were losing weight; others ventured out after they reached their goal. (Only a small percentage opt for no sweets or desserts.)

This week, think about *your* treat foods and tell yourself you don't need to feel guilty about wanting them—and having them.

**Make a list of the special foods that you do not want
to give up for the rest of your life:**

_____

_____

_____

_____

_____

*"If I want chocolate, I no longer try to put off the
feeling by ignoring it or trying to eat something else instead.
I found that I was eating too much other stuff, and when
I would finally 'break down,' I would eat too much."*

—*Ann Rae A. (100 pounds, 4 years)*

Goal(s) for this week: _____

_____

_____

Anticipated Obstacles   **Possible Solutions**

_____   _____

_____   _____

_____   _____

Exercise Plan

Monday: _____

Tuesday: _____

Wednesday: _____

Thursday: _____

Friday: _____

Saturday: _____

Sunday: _____

Try This for a Snack

❖ ⅔ cup chocolate chip cookie dough "lite" ice cream in a plain cone.

Calories: 200   Fat: 5 grams   (Marlene R.)

What I Ate: ———————— Monday ————————

MORNING   AFTERNOON   EVENING

Exercise / Accomplishments:

What I Ate: ———————— Tuesday ————————

MORNING   AFTERNOON   EVENING

Exercise / Accomplishments:

What I Ate: ———————— Wednesday ————————

MORNING   AFTERNOON   EVENING

Exercise / Accomplishments:

What I Ate: ———————— Thursday ————————

MORNING   AFTERNOON   EVENING

Exercise / Accomplishments:

What I Ate: ———————— Friday ————————

MORNING   AFTERNOON   EVENING

Exercise / Accomplishments:

What I Ate: ———————— Saturday ————————

MORNING   AFTERNOON   EVENING

Exercise / Accomplishments:

What I Ate: ———————— Sunday ————————

MORNING   AFTERNOON   EVENING

Exercise / Accomplishments:

———————— What Really Helped This Week: ————————

Develop a way to control tempting foods.

*"I don't have problem foods in the house—I go out for them.
As W. C. Fields said, 'I can resist anything except temptation!' "*

—**Bob W. (246 pounds, 23 years)**

A S IMPORTANT AS IT IS TO ALLOW YOURSELF OCCASIONAL treats, it's also important to accept that there will *never* be a time at which you can eat whatever you want, whenever you want. How can you learn to control your tempting foods?

It can help if you triage, grouping them into categories depending on the degree to which you feel you can control them. All of the masters take steps to control their highest-temptation items. Most just don't keep them around the house.

You may be able to eat other tempting items in controlled situations—say, in a restaurant or if you're in the presence of other people. You can also let packaging act as the controller, buying treats in single-serving sizes.

My don't-even-start foods:

_____

_____

My controlled-situation foods:
(List your tempting foods and how you can control them.)

_____

_____

_____

_____

Goal(s) for this week: _____

_____

_____

Anticipated Obstacles   **Possible Solutions**

_____   _____

_____   _____

_____   _____

Exercise Plan

Monday: _____

Tuesday: _____

Wednesday: _____

Thursday: _____

Friday: _____

Saturday: _____

Sunday: _____

Try This for Breakfast

❖ ½ cup cooked oatmeal (made with skim milk) mixed with ½ cup nonfat sugar-free vanilla pudding ❖ 1 slice reduced-calorie toast spread with 1 teaspoon reduced-fat peanut butter and 1 teaspoon honey.

Calories: 281   **Fat: 4 grams**   (Cindy F.)

What I Ate: —————————— Monday ——————————

MORNING   AFTERNOON   EVENING

Exercise / Accomplishments:

What I Ate: —————————— Tuesday ——————————

MORNING   AFTERNOON   EVENING

Exercise / Accomplishments:

What I Ate: —————————— Wednesday ——————————

MORNING   AFTERNOON   EVENING

Exercise / Accomplishments:

What I Ate: —————————— Thursday ——————————

MORNING   AFTERNOON   EVENING

Exercise / Accomplishments:

What I Ate: ———————— Friday ————————

MORNING   AFTERNOON   EVENING

Exercise / Accomplishments:

What I Ate: ———————— Saturday ————————

MORNING   AFTERNOON   EVENING

Exercise / Accomplishments:

What I Ate: ———————— Sunday ————————

MORNING   AFTERNOON   EVENING

Exercise / Accomplishments:

———————— What Really Helped This Week: ————————

Use behavior-modification strategies.

"When I was heavy, I ate what was on my plate and anything that was left over, including what was left on my children's plates. Now I eat from a small plate, and I've learned to scrape leftovers into the garbage disposal instead of eating them myself."

—*Patsy K. (99 pounds, 19 years)*

YOU'VE PROBABLY HEARD about all those behavior-modification tips, like using a small plate, putting down your fork between bites, eating slowly and not eating in front of the TV. But do they really work? According to the masters, some of them do, some don't—all depending on the person.

This week, make a concerted effort to test some of the masters' strategies. Check the ones that help:

_____Use smaller dishes and plates so that serving sizes seem larger.

_____Try hard to eat more slowly, putting your fork or spoon down between bites and chewing well before taking the next bite.

_____If you feel like having seconds, wait 20 minutes to see if the urge passes.

_____Don't eat with any distractions, like watching television or reading.

_____Don't eat any other place than at the table.

_____Find a symbolic way to finish a meal, like having a hot beverage, brushing your teeth or eating a mint.

_____Immediately put leftovers away or dispose of them.

If you find something that works, write it down here and on a notecard and post it where you'll regularly see it:

_____

Goal(s) for this week: _____

_____

_____

Anticipated Obstacles	Possible Solutions
_____	_____
_____	_____
_____	_____

Exercise Plan

Monday: _____

Tuesday: _____

Wednesday: _____

Thursday: _____

Friday: _____

Saturday: _____

Sunday: _____

Try This for Lunch

❖ **Asparagus-Chicken Salad:** 3 ounces cooked boneless, skinless chicken breast (in strips) tossed with 1 medium tomato (sliced) and 10 fresh asparagus spears (steamed). Marinate in ¼ cup fat-free Italian dressing. ❖ 6 reduced-fat wheat crackers ❖ 8 ounces peach yogurt (nonfat, sweetened with aspartame).

Calories: 390   Fat: 5.5 grams   (Ann F.)

What I Ate: ——————— **Monday** ———————

MORNING   AFTERNOON   EVENING

Exercise / Accomplishments:

What I Ate: ——————— **Tuesday** ———————

MORNING   AFTERNOON   EVENING

Exercise / Accomplishments:

What I Ate: ——————— **Wednesday** ———————

MORNING   AFTERNOON   EVENING

Exercise / Accomplishments:

What I Ate: ——————— **Thursday** ———————

MORNING   AFTERNOON   EVENING

Exercise / Accomplishments:

What I Ate: —————— Friday ——————

MORNING   AFTERNOON   EVENING

Exercise / Accomplishments:

What I Ate: —————— Saturday ——————

MORNING   AFTERNOON   EVENING

Exercise / Accomplishments:

What I Ate: —————— Sunday ——————

MORNING   AFTERNOON   EVENING

Exercise / Accomplishments:

————— What Really Helped This Week: —————

Get rid of the diet mentality.

*"I do not consider myself 'on a diet.' I know I must keep eating
this way for the rest of my life to stay thin and healthy.
My eating habits have changed for life."*

—*Hazel U. (40 pounds, 6 years)*

WHETHER YOU LOSE WEIGHT BY FORMALLY DIETING or by
following a nondieting approach, at some point you have
to get rid of the "diet" mentality. The word "diet" is filled with negative connotations—all related to deprivation, denial and short-
term changes.

Most masters, on the other hand, do not view the changes they've
made as deprivation. When asked, "Do you feel as if you're dieting?"
nine out of ten answered "No." And in response to the question "Do
you enjoy food?" the overwhelming majority said "Yes." The masters
eat what they want and want what they eat.

This week, any time you find yourself slipping into the "poor me"
mentality, remember: *You have made a choice to take control of your
weight in a healthful, positive way.*

**Make a list of the positive changes you've made or would like
to make that you feel you can live with for a lifetime**—for instance, eating breakfast, having five fruits and vegetables a day, using
a smaller plate for meals or walking every other day:

_____

_____

_____

_____

Goal(s) for this week: _____

_____

_____

Anticipated Obstacles   **Possible Solutions**

_____   _____

_____   _____

_____   _____

Exercise Plan

Monday: _____

Tuesday: _____

Wednesday: _____

Thursday: _____

Friday: _____

Saturday: _____

Sunday: _____

Try This for Supper

❖ 3 ounces broiled or grilled pork tenderloin ❖ ½ cup mashed
potatoes, made with skim milk ❖ 1 cup chopped broccoli,
sprinkled with 1 teaspoon grated Parmesan cheese ❖ **Sliced Fruit
Plate:** ½ each small apple, banana and pear ❖ 8 ounces skim milk.

Calories: 492   Fat: 9 grams   (Linda W.)

What I Ate: ———————— Monday ————————

MORNING   AFTERNOON   EVENING

Exercise / Accomplishments:

What I Ate: ———————— Tuesday ————————

MORNING   AFTERNOON   EVENING

Exercise / Accomplishments:

What I Ate: ———————— Wednesday ————————

MORNING   AFTERNOON   EVENING

Exercise / Accomplishments:

What I Ate: ———————— Thursday ————————

MORNING   AFTERNOON   EVENING

Exercise / Accomplishments:

What I Ate: ——————— **Friday** ———————

MORNING   AFTERNOON   EVENING

Exercise / Accomplishments:

What I Ate: ——————— **Saturday** ———————

MORNING   AFTERNOON   EVENING

Exercise / Accomplishments:

What I Ate: ——————— **Sunday** ———————

MORNING   AFTERNOON   EVENING

Exercise / Accomplishments:

——————— **What Really Helped This Week:** ———————

Prepare for the transition to maintenance.

*"It was trial and error. I watched the scale and went
by how my clothes fit. If I felt myself creeping back up,
I started to watch what I ate and exercised more.
I never let myself gain more than 5 pounds."*

—**Beth W.** *(73 pounds, 18 years)*

WHETHER YOU'RE ALREADY THERE or on your way, it's wise to start thinking about how you'll make the transition from the weight-loss stage to the keep-it-off-forever state of maintenance. The masters used the following techniques to make the transition.

Check the strategies that may be helpful to you:

____Eat more of what you're already eating. Experiment by slowly increasing amounts of foods.

____Let the scale guide you. Weigh yourself regularly to see if you're eating too much or too little.

____Get support. If you went to a program to lose weight, research suggests that sticking with it well into maintenance is critical for keeping the weight off.

____Add a few treats. Some masters who cut out sweets while losing added reasonable amounts back during maintenance.

____Get rid of your large-size clothes.

____Write down everything you eat.

____Balance food and exercise. Some masters used exercise when they ate a little too much.

Rest assured that the transition stage is not a hardship for everyone. *About 25 percent of the masters say that their food habits are no different during maintenance than when they were losing weight.*

Goal(s) for this week: _____

_____

_____

Anticipated Obstacles	**Possible Solutions**
_____	_____
_____	_____
_____	_____

Exercise Plan

Monday: _____

Tuesday: _____

Wednesday: _____

Thursday: _____

Friday: _____

Saturday: _____

Sunday: _____

Try This for Breakfast

❖ **Veggie Scramble:** Microwave or steam 1 cup mixed vegetables (chopped broccoli, onion, green pepper, mushrooms). Scramble with 1 whole egg, 1 egg white, ¼ cup skim milk and 1 slice (¾ ounce) crumbled low-fat cheese in a nonstick skillet. ❖ 6 ounces orange juice.

Calories: 295   **Fat: 9.5 grams**   **(Joe K.)**

What I Ate: ——————— Monday ———————

MORNING   AFTERNOON   EVENING

Exercise / Accomplishments:

What I Ate: ——————— Tuesday ———————

MORNING   AFTERNOON   EVENING

Exercise / Accomplishments:

What I Ate: ——————— Wednesday ———————

MORNING   AFTERNOON   EVENING

Exercise / Accomplishments:

What I Ate: ——————— Thursday ———————

MORNING   AFTERNOON   EVENING

Exercise / Accomplishments:

What I Ate: —————————— Friday ——————————

MORNING   AFTERNOON   EVENING

Exercise / Accomplishments:

What I Ate: —————————— Saturday ——————————

MORNING   AFTERNOON   EVENING

Exercise / Accomplishments:

What I Ate: —————————— Sunday ——————————

MORNING   AFTERNOON   EVENING

Exercise / Accomplishments:

—————————— What Really Helped This Week: ——————————

III

Getting a New Food Life

Learning How
to Eat Like the Masters

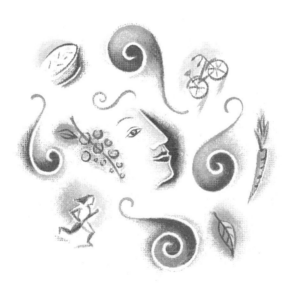

Eat "Large."

"When, instead of my customary rib-eye steak, I ate a skinless chicken breast or halibut steak, I discovered that I could eat twice as much food for the same calorie level. And when, instead of four or five slices of pizza with sausage, I ate two slices of my own vegetarian pizza with a big salad, I could get full on a lot less calories. I figured out how to 'eat large.'"

—Stan J. (103 pounds, 5 years)

SOME OF THE BEST NEWS FROM THE MASTERS is that if you want to get a new food life, you don't have to go around hungry all the time. They have learned how to get the most for their calories by finding foods that will fill them up but are not fattening.

Many did a bit of homework to learn which foods have fat in them and which don't. In the beginning, some masters found it was easier to keep meals simple—choosing, for instance, a baked potato, salad with fat-free dressing, a skinless baked chicken breast with herbs and a piece of fruit. From there, they branched out.

This week, get a book that lists calories and fat grams for individual portions of foods. Read labels, too. Keep a running log in your food diary of calories (and fat grams, if desired) in every item you eat.

List some foods you like that give you the largest portion sizes for their calorie level:

_____   _____

_____   _____

_____   _____

Goal(s) for this week: _____

_____

_____

Anticipated Obstacles	Possible Solutions
_____	_____
_____	_____
_____	_____

Exercise Plan

Monday: _____

Tuesday: _____

Wednesday: _____

Thursday: _____

Friday: _____

Saturday: _____

Sunday: _____

Try This for Lunch

❖ **Tuna Salad Sandwich:** 2 slices whole wheat bread spread with 3 ounces water-packed tuna mixed with 1½ tablespoons fat-free mayonnaise and 2 teaspoons sweet-pickle relish ❖ 1 carrot cut into strips and dipped into 1 tablespoon fat-free ranch dressing ❖ 1 large plum.

Calories: 394   **Fat: 4.5 grams**   (Lorraine W.)

Weekly Diary

What I Ate: ——————— **Monday** ———————

MORNING   AFTERNOON   EVENING

Exercise / Accomplishments:

What I Ate: ——————— **Tuesday** ———————

MORNING   AFTERNOON   EVENING

Exercise / Accomplishments:

What I Ate: ——————— **Wednesday** ———————

MORNING   AFTERNOON   EVENING

Exercise / Accomplishments:

What I Ate: ——————— **Thursday** ———————

MORNING   AFTERNOON   EVENING

Exercise / Accomplishments:

What I Ate: —————— Friday ——————

MORNING   AFTERNOON   EVENING

Exercise / Accomplishments:

What I Ate: —————— Saturday ——————

MORNING   AFTERNOON   EVENING

Exercise / Accomplishments:

What I Ate: —————— Sunday ——————

MORNING   AFTERNOON   EVENING

Exercise / Accomplishments:

—————— What Really Helped This Week: ——————

Be consistent.

*"When I was hungry, I used to eat all the time.
It didn't matter if I had just finished dinner
30 minutes before. Now I try to eat three
meals a day and limit my snacks."*

—*Peppi S. (27 pounds, 9 years)*

D O YOU EAT BREAKFAST? Are you a lunch-skipper? The masters no longer eat haphazardly. They go out of their way to enjoy regular meals.

A number stress the importance of having breakfast. Evidence suggests that people who sit down to breakfast indulge in fewer impulsive snacks throughout the day and eat more balanced meals.

While most masters enjoy three meals a day, with planned snacks in between, some are grazers. Diane J. says, "I try to eat something at least every three hours so I am never superhungry."

You need to develop a daily routine—one that gives you consistency in your eating habits.

This week, sit down and eat at least two well-balanced meals each day (preferably three). Each one should include some low-fat protein (chicken, fish or low-fat cheese), vegetables, fruit and a grain or two. If you skip breakfast, have a little something each morning—a bowl of cereal with skim milk, a low-fat milkshake (made in a blender with a cup of skim milk, a frozen banana and a teaspoon of vanilla extract), a piece of toast and a small glass of juice, a yogurt or an English muffin and a piece of fruit.

*"Eating breakfast is a big change and
is essential to keep me on track."*

—*Joanne F. (80 pounds, 8 years)*

Goal(s) for this week: _____

_____

_____

Anticipated Obstacles   Possible Solutions

_____   _____

_____   _____

_____   _____

Exercise Plan

Monday: _____

Tuesday: _____

Wednesday: _____

Thursday: _____

Friday: _____

Saturday: _____

Sunday: _____

Try This for Supper

❖ **Seafood Chef's Salad:** 3 cups Boston lettuce, 3 ounces cooked

fish (tuna, cod, halibut), ⅓ cup broccoli florets, 4 cherry tomatoes,

1 medium carrot (shredded), 2 tablespoons vinaigrette dressing

❖ 2 (1-ounce) slices warm French bread ❖ 8 ounces skim milk.

Calories: 500   Fat: 9 grams   (Jane Brody)

What I Ate: ———————— Monday ————————————

MORNING   AFTERNOON   EVENING

Exercise / Accomplishments:

What I Ate: ———————— Tuesday ————————————

MORNING   AFTERNOON   EVENING

Exercise / Accomplishments:

What I Ate: ———————— Wednesday————————

MORNING   AFTERNOON   EVENING

Exercise / Accomplishments:

What I Ate: ———————— Thursday ————————————

MORNING   AFTERNOON   EVENING

Exercise / Accomplishments:

What I Ate: ———————— Friday ————————

MORNING   AFTERNOON   EVENING

Exercise / Accomplishments:

What I Ate: ———————— Saturday ————————

MORNING   AFTERNOON   EVENING

Exercise / Accomplishments:

What I Ate: ———————— Sunday ————————

MORNING   AFTERNOON   EVENING

Exercise / Accomplishments:

———————— What Really Helped This Week: ————————

Little by little, shave the fat.

"To begin a low-fat diet, start changing things you eat little by little. Instead of eating a doughnut for breakfast, eat a bagel. Instead of spaghetti with cream sauce, try a tomato-based sauce. It takes some time."

—Debbie T. (62 pounds, 6 years)

WHEN ASKED THE THREE MOST IMPORTANT FACTORS in keeping their weight down, the number-one food-related response from the masters was "watch my fat intake." Chuck B. says, "You'll find it tastes *better*."

How do you go about eating low-fat? The masters do the obvious—choose baked and broiled foods over fried versions, nonfat and low-fat dairy products over whole-milk products and low-fat baked goods like bread and English muffins over breakfast pastries and rich desserts. The most significant way they cut fat, in the words of Mabel H., is to "refrain from using visible fats—butter, margarine, salad dressings, cream."

This week, cut back on added fats by trying the following:

❖ For one or two days, circle or highlight on your food diary all the "added" fats you eat, noting the exact amount. Then, for the rest of the week, try to cut your added fat intake at least in half.

❖ Try two or three reduced-fat or fat-free fats—for instance, margarine, butter, mayonnaise, cream cheese or sour cream.

"I never feel deprived. Now, I just don't like the feeling of greasy, fatty foods."

—Carole C. (40 pounds, 20 years)

Weekly Forecast

Goal(s) for this week: _____

_____

_____

Anticipated Obstacles   Possible Solutions

_____   _____

_____   _____

_____   _____

Exercise Plan

Monday: _____

Tuesday: _____

Wednesday: _____

Thursday: _____

Friday: _____

Saturday: _____

Sunday: _____

Try This for Breakfast

❖ 2 low-fat buttermilk pancakes, topped with 2 teaspoons nonfat margarine and 2 tablespoons real maple syrup ❖ ½ small pear (sliced).

Calories: 300   Fat: 4 grams   (Don Mauer)

What I Ate: ———————— Monday ————————————

MORNING   AFTERNOON   EVENING

Exercise / Accomplishments:

What I Ate: ———————— Tuesday ————————————

MORNING   AFTERNOON   EVENING

Exercise / Accomplishments:

What I Ate: ———————— Wednesday ————————

MORNING   AFTERNOON   EVENING

Exercise / Accomplishments:

What I Ate: ———————— Thursday ————————————

MORNING   AFTERNOON   EVENING

Exercise / Accomplishments:

Friday

What I Ate:

MORNING   AFTERNOON   EVENING

Exercise / Accomplishments:

Saturday

What I Ate:

MORNING   AFTERNOON   EVENING

Exercise / Accomplishments:

Sunday

What I Ate:

MORNING   AFTERNOON   EVENING

Exercise / Accomplishments:

What Really Helped This Week:

Find new ways to enjoy vegetables and fruits.

"I eat average portions of foods.
If I still feel hungry after giving myself time to feel full,
I take seconds of vegetables.
They didn't get me up to 335 pounds!"

—*Emil R. (115 pounds, 9 years)*

MOST MASTERS EAT VEGETABLES at least two or three times a day, and many enjoy fruits just as frequently. Salads seem to factor into masters' meal planning in a big way, probably because lettuce and other greens are so filling and almost calorie-free. But beware the dressing (a small ladle can easily scoop up several hundred calories worth).

This week, try at least three of the following tips for enlivening your meals with more vegetables and fruits:

❖ Try two or three new fruits or vegetables. Switch from the old familiar green beans and bananas to okra, winter squash and kiwi.

❖ Eat a few "meal" salads, starting with greens and chopped vegetables as the base, but tossing in several ounces of cooked chicken, turkey, low-fat cheese and/or legumes.

❖ Put fruit in your vegetables. Add sliced or chopped apples, pears, grapes, melon, kiwi and orange sections to tossed spinach and cabbage salads.

❖ Have at least one fruit serving with each meal.

❖ Experiment with nonfat flavorings, such as nutmeg and lemon juice on spinach and broccoli or dill weed and Dijon mustard on green beans.

❖ Mix your vegetables. Combine corn and beans; zucchini with onions and tomatoes; red potato and carrot slivers.

Goal(s) for this week: _____

_____

_____

Anticipated Obstacles	**Possible Solutions**
_____	_____
_____	_____
_____	_____

Exercise Plan

Monday: _____

Tuesday: _____

Wednesday: _____

Thursday: _____

Friday: _____

Saturday: _____

Sunday: _____

Try This for Lunch

❖ **Tuna-Pasta Salad:** Mix 2 ounces (drained) water-pack albacore tuna, 1 cup cooked corkscrew pasta, 1 cup thawed frozen vegetables (broccoli, cauliflower, carrots, peas), 1 small chopped tomato, 1 cup endive. Toss with 1 tablespoon grated Parmesan cheese ❖ ½ cup raspberries (unsweetened).

| Calories: 399 | Fat: 5 grams | (Patsy K.) |

Monday

What I Ate: ———————

MORNING   AFTERNOON   EVENING

Exercise / Accomplishments:

Tuesday

What I Ate: ———————

MORNING   AFTERNOON   EVENING

Exercise / Accomplishments:

Wednesday

What I Ate: ———————

MORNING   AFTERNOON   EVENING

Exercise / Accomplishments:

Thursday

What I Ate: ———————

MORNING   AFTERNOON   EVENING

Exercise / Accomplishments:

What I Ate: ——————— Friday ———————

MORNING   AFTERNOON   EVENING

Exercise / Accomplishments:

What I Ate: ——————— Saturday ———————

MORNING   AFTERNOON   EVENING

Exercise / Accomplishments:

What I Ate: ——————— Sunday ———————

MORNING   AFTERNOON   EVENING

Exercise / Accomplishments:

——————— What Really Helped This Week: ———————

Go for grains.

*"Knowing that I could have generous amounts of carbohydrates,
fruits and vegetables in exchange for fat put me on the road to
weight loss. It's a whole new world being normal in size
and not having to worry about gaining weight again."*

—*Virginia L. (97 pounds, 4 years)*

TAKE IT FROM THE MASTERS: Grains should be the mainstay
of your diet when you're watching your weight. Grain-based
foods will not make you fat unless you eat too much of them or
you load them up with butter, margarine and sour cream.

Go for whole-grain versions whenever possible. Some studies
have shown that high-fiber foods eaten at breakfast or lunch signif-
icantly reduce the amount consumed at the next meal. Shift away
from higher-fat items like regular muffins, quick breads, oily crackers and doughnuts.

**To work in grains without the fat this week,
try the following:**

❖ Have two servings with each meal—say, an ounce of whole
grain cereal and a slice of rye toast with jelly for breakfast, a sandwich with two slices of whole wheat bread for lunch; ½ cup of pasta
with a slice of warm Italian bread for supper.

❖ Take at least three grain foods that you normally have with fat
and try them without.

❖ Have sandwiches with fancy mustard or fat-free mayonnaise
instead of regular mayonnaise.

Goal(s) for this week: _____

_____

_____

Anticipated Obstacles   Possible Solutions

_____   _____

_____   _____

_____   _____

Exercise Plan

Monday: _____

Tuesday: _____

Wednesday: _____

Thursday: _____

Friday: _____

Saturday: _____

Sunday: _____

Try This for Supper

❖ **Southwestern Lasagna:** 3 ounces cooked lasagna noodles (1½ noodles) layered with ½ cup nonfat cottage cheese, ⅓ cup salsa and 1 ounce shredded reduced-fat Monterey Jack cheese ❖ **Garlic Breadstick:** 1-ounce breadstick sprayed with butter-flavored nonstick spray and sprinkled with garlic salt ❖ 1 cup steamed snap peas.

Calories: 500   Fat: 9 grams   (Mary Ann K.)

What I Ate: —————— Monday ——————

MORNING   AFTERNOON   EVENING

Exercise / Accomplishments:

What I Ate: —————— Tuesday ——————

MORNING   AFTERNOON   EVENING

Exercise / Accomplishments:

What I Ate: —————— Wednesday ——————

MORNING   AFTERNOON   EVENING

Exercise / Accomplishments:

What I Ate: —————— Thursday ——————

MORNING   AFTERNOON   EVENING

Exercise / Accomplishments:

What I Ate: ———————— Friday ————————

MORNING   AFTERNOON   EVENING

Exercise / Accomplishments:

What I Ate: ———————— Saturday ————————

MORNING   AFTERNOON   EVENING

Exercise / Accomplishments:

What I Ate: ———————— Sunday ————————

MORNING   AFTERNOON   EVENING

Exercise / Accomplishments:

———————— What Really Helped This Week: ————————

Lighten up on meats.

*"I stopped eating a lot of meat and concentrated
on vegetables, fruits, fish, chicken and cottage cheese.
I never would have dreamed that cutting out meat
would make such a difference."*

—*Susan C. (105 pounds, 16 years)*

O VER AND OVER, THE MASTERS SURPRISED ME by talking about how little meat they eat. And when they do have it, they generally favor light-colored "meats"—namely poultry and seafood, which also tend to be light in fat and calories.

You don't have to eliminate red meats completely. Linda M. says, "I use meat as a condiment." Portion sizes are what trip many people up. While the standard for many steak lovers is 8 to 12 ounces, the recommended portion for meats, poultry and seafood is just 2 to 3 ounces (no bigger than a deck of cards) of cooked food, without bones, skin and fat. Two daily servings are plenty.

Here are some goals for the week:

❖ Weigh meats on a food scale, after cooking, to check your portion sizes.

❖ If you're a red-meat eater, have fish, shellfish or skinless breast of chicken or turkey in place of meat a minimum of three times this week.

❖ Have at least one serving of legumes (½ cup, cooked) as in vegetarian baked beans, or mixed with pasta and vegetables, or as part of a tossed salad or in a low-fat soup.

Goal(s) for this week: _____

_____

_____

Anticipated Obstacles	Possible Solutions
_____	_____
_____	_____
_____	_____

Exercise Plan

Monday: _____

Tuesday: _____

Wednesday: _____

Thursday: _____

Friday: _____

Saturday: _____

Sunday: _____

Try This for Supper

❖ 1¼ cups turkey or vegetarian chili, topped with 2 tablespoons nonfat sour cream and 1 ounce shredded reduced-fat cheddar cheese ❖ 10 baby carrots ❖ 5 unsalted saltines.

Calories: 496　　　　**Fat: 12.5 grams**　　　　(Julie J.)

What I Ate: ——— **Monday** ———

MORNING   AFTERNOON   EVENING

Exercise / Accomplishments:

What I Ate: ——— **Tuesday** ———

MORNING   AFTERNOON   EVENING

Exercise / Accomplishments:

What I Ate: ——— **Wednesday** ———

MORNING   AFTERNOON   EVENING

Exercise / Accomplishments:

What I Ate: ——— **Thursday** ———

MORNING   AFTERNOON   EVENING

Exercise / Accomplishments:

Friday

What I Ate:

MORNING   AFTERNOON   EVENING

Exercise / Accomplishments:

Saturday

What I Ate:

MORNING   AFTERNOON   EVENING

Exercise / Accomplishments:

Sunday

What I Ate:

MORNING   AFTERNOON   EVENING

Exercise / Accomplishments:

What Really Helped This Week:

Shift your dairy choices.

"I changed from whole milk and finally to nonfat.
I drank 2 percent until I started to like it and
then changed to nonfat months later."

—*Rosetta F. (25 pounds, 3 years)*

ACCORDING TO RECENT TASTE TESTS conducted by Center for Science in the Public Interest, few consumers are able to tell the difference between milk of varying fat levels.

If you drink whole milk instead of skim, you'll wind up with about 200 more calories and an extra 24 grams of fat for every 3 cups (the minimum needed to meet the calcium recommendation for most adults). Here's how the different types of milk stack up:

1 cup milk	calories	fat grams
skim	85	0
1%	100	2.5
2%	120	4.5
whole (3.5%)	150	8

Try the following techniques this week:

❖ Make the change gradually.

❖ Rather than using half-and-half in your coffee, try substituting fat-free half-and-half, evaporated skim milk or a mixture of half-and-half with skim or evaporated skim milk.

❖ Sample at least two or three kinds of fat-free and reduced-fat cheese to see which kinds you prefer. (An ounce and a half of cheese is considered a serving.)

❖ Try two or three new flavors of aspartame-sweetened yogurt. (One cup of yogurt is considered a serving.)

Weekly Forecast

Goal(s) for this week: _____

_____

_____

Anticipated Obstacles	Possible Solutions
_____	_____
_____	_____
_____	_____

Exercise Plan

Monday: _____

Tuesday: _____

Wednesday: _____

Thursday: _____

Friday: _____

Saturday: _____

Sunday: _____

Try This for Lunch

❖ 1 cup tomato soup (such as Campbell's Healthy Request)

❖ **Grilled Cheese Sandwich:** 2 slices rye bread, 2 slices (1½ ounces) fat-free American cheese. Grill in a nonstick skillet coated with nonstick butter-flavored spray. ❖ 8 ounces skim milk flavored with 1 teaspoon vanilla and 1 packet low-calorie sweetener, if desired.

| Calories: 379 | Fat: 4 grams | (Emil R.) |

What I Ate: ——————— Monday ———————

MORNING   AFTERNOON   EVENING

Exercise / Accomplishments:

What I Ate: ——————— Tuesday ———————

MORNING   AFTERNOON   EVENING

Exercise / Accomplishments:

What I Ate: ——————— Wednesday ———————

MORNING   AFTERNOON   EVENING

Exercise / Accomplishments:

What I Ate: ——————— Thursday ———————

MORNING   AFTERNOON   EVENING

Exercise / Accomplishments:

What I Ate: ——————— Friday ———————

MORNING   AFTERNOON   EVENING

Exercise / Accomplishments:

What I Ate: ——————— Saturday ———————

MORNING   AFTERNOON   EVENING

Exercise / Accomplishments:

What I Ate: ——————— Sunday ———————

MORNING   AFTERNOON   EVENING

Exercise / Accomplishments:

——————— What Really Helped This Week: ———————

Learn to cook a new way.

"Everything is about taste.
We can be satisfied with fewer fat grams if the food tastes good."

—Diane J. (43 pounds, 5 years)

IT CAN SEEM DAUNTING to learn how to cook a new way, but you can do it in "baby steps," says Diane J. Her philosophy is, "You take out, you put back in." When she takes oil out of baked goods, for instance, she adds back moisture in the form of applesauce or crushed pineapple. (Each tablespoon of fat that you cut out will save about 100 calories and at least 11 grams of fat.)

Brad H. advises, "Learn five new low-fat recipes, and cook them instead of your favorites."

To move yourself in the right direction, try the following:

❖ Take a minimum of two of your favorite recipes and cut back the amount of fat by at least one half. In baked goods, you can substitute pureed fruit (baby food works fine), prunes or applesauce for the fat you remove. Next time, see if you can cut the fat further.

❖ Buy one low-fat cookbook or magazine and try a few new recipes.

❖ Treat yourself to some special fat-free seasonings—fresh basil or butter flavoring for vegetables, fancy mustard for raw vegetables, pure vanilla extract rather than imitation, peppercorns in a new pepper mill.

"You have to zero in on the foods you've always loved.
Then go out and find low-fat and low-sugar
alternatives to them."

—JoAnna L. (130 pounds, 3 years)

Goal(s) for this week: _____

_____

_____

Anticipated Obstacles   **Possible Solutions**

_____   _____

_____   _____

_____   _____

Exercise Plan

Monday: _____

Tuesday: _____

Wednesday: _____

Thursday: _____

Friday: _____

Saturday: _____

Sunday: _____

Try This for Breakfast

❖ **French Toast:** 2 slices reduced-calorie whole wheat bread dipped in a mixture of ¼ cup egg substitute, 1 teaspoon vanilla extract, 1 packet low-calorie sweetener and 2 tablespoons skim milk. Cook in a nonstick skillet sprayed with butter-flavored spray and top with 2 tablespoons reduced-calorie pancake syrup. ❖ 1 slice honeydew melon.

Calories: 286   **Fat: 3.5 grams**   (David D.)

Weekly Diary

Monday

What I Ate:

MORNING   AFTERNOON   EVENING

Exercise / Accomplishments:

Tuesday

What I Ate:

MORNING   AFTERNOON   EVENING

Exercise / Accomplishments:

Wednesday

What I Ate:

MORNING   AFTERNOON   EVENING

Exercise / Accomplishments:

Thursday

What I Ate:

MORNING   AFTERNOON   EVENING

Exercise / Accomplishments:

What I Ate: ——————— Friday ———————

MORNING   AFTERNOON   EVENING

Exercise / Accomplishments:

What I Ate: ——————— Saturday ———————

MORNING   AFTERNOON   EVENING

Exercise / Accomplishments:

What I Ate: ——————— Sunday ———————

MORNING   AFTERNOON   EVENING

Exercise / Accomplishments:

——————— What Really Helped This Week: ———————

Be patient with your taste buds.

*"I prefer not to slap butter on my potato,
and I eat no fried foods or cream sauces.
If I throw pork chops or chicken breasts in the oven,
it's with lemon, some parsley and onions.
I absolutely prefer to eat this way."*

—*Lynda C. (41 pounds, 6 years)*

HOW DO YOU REACH THE POINT where, like the masters, you actually develop a *preference* for low-fat foods? In the words of Vicki B., "It takes a little while to adjust."

**To help yourself acquire a taste for low-fat eating,
try the following mind games of some of the masters:**

❖ Joanna M. advises, "When you're tempted to eat something high-fat, think about a place on your body that you wish were thinner and remember how easily the body stores fat because it's already in the right form."

❖ When Ann Q. is tempted to eat something high in fat, she thinks "heart attack on a plate" or pictures an unappetizing layer of lard sitting on top of the treat.

Eventually, if you stick with it, you will reach a point where, like the masters, you *prefer your new way of eating to your old.*

Goal(s) for this week: _____

_____

_____

Anticipated Obstacles   **Possible Solutions**

_____   _____

_____   _____

_____   _____

Exercise Plan

Monday: _____

Tuesday: _____

Wednesday: _____

Thursday: _____

Friday: _____

Saturday: _____

Sunday: _____

Try This for a Snack

❖ **Curried Popcorn:** 4 cups air-popped popcorn tossed with ½ tablespoon olive oil and seasoned with curry powder and salt.

Calories: 185   Fat: 8 grams   (Gail O.)

30

What I Ate: ——————— **Monday** ———————

MORNING   AFTERNOON   EVENING

Exercise / Accomplishments:

What I Ate: ——————— **Tuesday** ———————

MORNING   AFTERNOON   EVENING

Exercise / Accomplishments:

What I Ate: ——————— **Wednesday** ———————

MORNING   AFTERNOON   EVENING

Exercise / Accomplishments:

What I Ate: ——————— **Thursday** ———————

MORNING   AFTERNOON   EVENING

Exercise / Accomplishments:

What I Ate: ——————— Friday ———————

MORNING   AFTERNOON   EVENING

Exercise / Accomplishments:

What I Ate: ——————— Saturday ———————

MORNING   AFTERNOON   EVENING

Exercise / Accomplishments:

What I Ate: ——————— Sunday ———————

MORNING   AFTERNOON   EVENING

Exercise / Accomplishments:

——————— What Really Helped This Week: ———————

Figure out if your "full button" needs fixing.

*"In the old days, when I was learning how to eat healthy,
I would not have stopped until my plate was clean. I can now
hear that inner voice telling me when I've had enough."*

—*JoAnna L. (130 pounds, 3 years)*

WOULDN'T IT BE NICE if we could all simply eat when we're hungry and stop when we're full? The truth is that many of us don't really know when to cut ourselves off and eat beyond the point of being full.

This week, see if you can pay better attention to your body's internal hunger cues. Tell yourself, as Jennifer P. does, that it is OK to stop eating when you "feel satisfied, not *stuffed*."

Here are some tips:

❖ Don't let yourself get too hungry. When you're ravenous, you may find yourself eating too much food too fast.

❖ Put half to three quarters of the amount of food you usually eat on your plate. Have seconds only if you are truly hungry.

❖ After you're about halfway through your meal—or before you decide you want second helpings—pause and wait for 15 to 20 minutes.

❖ To break yourself of the plate-cleaning habit, practice leaving some food on your plate after each meal.

❖ Find a symbolic way to tell your body, "Meal's over." Jennie C. brushes her teeth to get that "finished-with-food feeling."

Goal(s) for this week: _____

_____

_____

Anticipated Obstacles	Possible Solutions
_____	_____
_____	_____
_____	_____

Exercise Plan

Monday: _____

Tuesday: _____

Wednesday: _____

Thursday: _____

Friday: _____

Saturday: _____

Sunday: _____

Try This for Breakfast

❖ ½ medium cantaloupe ❖ 1 egg scrambled with ¼ cup sliced mushrooms, plus chives and basil, topped with 3 tablespoons salsa ❖ 1 slice whole wheat toast with 2 teaspoons apricot preserves.

Calories: 300   Fat: 7.5 grams   (Lynda M.)

What I Ate: ———————— Monday ————————

MORNING   AFTERNOON   EVENING

Exercise / Accomplishments:

What I Ate: ———————— Tuesday ————————

MORNING   AFTERNOON   EVENING

Exercise / Accomplishments:

What I Ate: ———————— Wednesday ————————

MORNING   AFTERNOON   EVENING

Exercise / Accomplishments:

What I Ate: ———————— Thursday ————————

MORNING   AFTERNOON   EVENING

Exercise / Accomplishments:

Friday

What I Ate:

MORNING   AFTERNOON   EVENING

Exercise / Accomplishments:

Saturday

What I Ate:

MORNING   AFTERNOON   EVENING

Exercise / Accomplishments:

Sunday

What I Ate:

MORNING   AFTERNOON   EVENING

Exercise / Accomplishments:

What Really Helped This Week:

Learn what a reasonable portion size is.

*"Because I don't know when to stop eating,
I must decide in advance how much I'm going to have.
If I sit down with a box of graham crackers, I could eat a whole
packet. Likewise with frozen yogurt. So I set an amount
ahead of time: two crackers, one bar of frozen yogurt."*

—*Jane Brody (32 pounds, 26 years)*

T HE MASTERS GO OUT OF THEIR WAY to limit portion sizes by serving themselves finite amounts. But many people have little clue what a "normal" size is. Several studies suggest that overweight individuals are particularly likely to report eating less food than they've actually consumed. Being off in your estimate can add up, and calorie books don't necessarily list "typical" portion sizes that you find on the market.

This week, make a concerted effort to weigh and measure every calorie-containing item you eat. (To do this, you'll need a decent food scale, a set of measuring spoons and a set of measuring cups.) To guide your portion sizes for various foods, go by the amount listed for a single serving on package labels.

Consider buying foods in single-portion amounts (especially tempting items). Patsy K. says, "I use a small plate, a small bowl and a small cup."

The good news is that you need not be a fanatic food weigher and measurer for the rest of your life. With time, you'll likely be able to gauge amounts by eyeballing. Indeed, most masters stop measuring once they get the hang of judging proper portion sizes.

Goal(s) for this week: _____

_____

_____

Anticipated Obstacles	Possible Solutions
_____	_____
_____	_____
_____	_____

Exercise Plan

Monday: _____

Tuesday: _____

Wednesday: _____

Thursday: _____

Friday: _____

Saturday: _____

Sunday: _____

Try This for Lunch

❖ **Vegetarian Sandwich:** 2 slices pumpernickel bread, ¼ cup each shredded carrots and mung bean sprouts, 2 slices (1½ ounces) fat-free American cheese, 2 teaspoons sunflower seeds, 1½ tablespoons fat-free mayonnaise ❖ 10 fat-free tortilla chips with ¼ cup salsa.

Calories: 392   Fat: 6 grams   (Randy W.)

WEEK

32

What I Ate: ——————— Monday ———————

MORNING   AFTERNOON   EVENING

Exercise / Accomplishments:

What I Ate: ——————— Tuesday ———————

MORNING   AFTERNOON   EVENING

Exercise / Accomplishments:

What I Ate: ——————— Wednesday ———————

MORNING   AFTERNOON   EVENING

Exercise / Accomplishments:

What I Ate: ——————— Thursday ———————

MORNING   AFTERNOON   EVENING

Exercise / Accomplishments:

WEEK

32

Friday

What I Ate:

MORNING   AFTERNOON   EVENING

Exercise / Accomplishments:

Saturday

What I Ate:

MORNING   AFTERNOON   EVENING

Exercise / Accomplishments:

Sunday

What I Ate:

MORNING   AFTERNOON   EVENING

Exercise / Accomplishments:

What Really Helped This Week:

Plan ahead.

*"My wife and I plan our suppers a week ahead—
we have a fixed menu six out of seven nights. The seventh
night is 'wild-card night,' when we'll try something new
from a low-fat cookbook or magazine."*

—*Don Mauer (113 pounds, 5 years)*

WHEN I ASKED THE MASTERS, "What determines how much
you eat at any one meal or snack?" their most common responses had to do with *planning ahead*. Most plan day-to-day meals
ahead of time—sometimes up to a week in advance.

It's much easier to eat carelessly when your resistance is low and
you haven't planned ahead. On the other hand, if your refrigerator
is stocked with fresh fruits and vegetables and you have thawed some
chicken overnight, you're far more likely to eat healthfully.

You don't have to plan every detail as long as you're well sup-
plied with fruits, vegetables and low-fat carbohydrate foods. "The
important thing is that you're not caught off guard so that in a
weak moment you can justify why you're going to eat something,"
says Kay D.

**This week, sit down on Saturday or Sunday and map out
your evening meals for the week ahead:**

_____

_____

_____

_____

_____

_____

Goal(s) for this week: _____

_____

_____

Anticipated Obstacles   **Possible Solutions**

_____   _____

_____   _____

_____   _____

Exercise Plan

Monday: _____

Tuesday: _____

Wednesday: _____

Thursday: _____

Friday: _____

Saturday: _____

Sunday: _____

Try This for Supper

❖ 4 ounces grilled swordfish ❖ 1 medium baked potato (4 ounces) with 2 tablespoons fat-free Peppercorn Ranch dressing ❖ 1 cup steamed spinach with ¼ cup diced tomatoes ❖ 1 cup shredded carrots with 1 tablespoon raisins mixed with 2 tablespoons fat-free French dressing and low-calorie sweetener to taste.

Calories: 485   **Fat: 7.5 grams**   (Pat C.)

What I Ate: —————————— Monday ——————————

MORNING   AFTERNOON   EVENING

Exercise / Accomplishments:

What I Ate: —————————— Tuesday ——————————

MORNING   AFTERNOON   EVENING

Exercise / Accomplishments:

What I Ate: —————————— Wednesday ——————————

MORNING   AFTERNOON   EVENING

Exercise / Accomplishments:

What I Ate: —————————— Thursday ——————————

MORNING   AFTERNOON   EVENING

Exercise / Accomplishments:

What I Ate: —————— **Friday** ——————

MORNING   AFTERNOON   EVENING

Exercise / Accomplishments:

What I Ate: —————— **Saturday** ——————

MORNING   AFTERNOON   EVENING

Exercise / Accomplishments:

What I Ate: —————— **Sunday** ——————

MORNING   AFTERNOON   EVENING

Exercise / Accomplishments:

—————— **What Really Helped This Week:** ——————

Remember: A low-fat portion
is still a portion.

*"I have found that fat-free desserts do not work for me.
I think it might be that word 'FREE'—I see it and I think
it means free to eat as much as I want of it."*

—*Patsy K. (99 pounds, 19 years)*

TAKE IT FROM THE MASTERS WHO LEARNED THE HARD WAY: Being mindful of portions is important even when those portions are low-fat or fat-free.

The truth is that foods with little or no fat do provide calories. Sometimes reduced-fat products have as many or nearly as many calories as their regular counterparts.

The low-fat label may also trick you into eating more throughout the day. A study reported in the *Journal of the American Dietetic Association* showed that women who were given yogurt labeled "low fat" before a buffet ate more calories during that meal than when they got yogurt that had about the same calories but was labeled "high fat."

Given two products with the same or a similar number of calories, it *is* usually healthier to choose the one with less fat. Just don't kid yourself that you can eat all you want and keep your weight down.

This week, when you're in the supermarket, make it a point to compare reduced-fat products with their regular counterparts to see if there really is a significant calorie difference. Check items like candies, baked goods, ice cream, cookies, salty snack foods and peanut butter.

Goal(s) for this week: _____

_____

Anticipated Obstacles   **Possible Solutions**

_____   _____

_____   _____

_____   _____

Exercise Plan

Monday: _____

Tuesday: _____

Wednesday: _____

Thursday: _____

Friday: _____

Saturday: _____

Sunday: _____

Try This for Breakfast

❖ **Breakfast Shake:** Whir in a blender until smooth 6 ounces strawberry yogurt (nonfat, sweetened with aspartame), 1 medium banana, 1 tablespoon wheat germ, ⅓ cup skim milk, ¼ cup orange juice.

Calories: 270   **Fat: 1.5 grams**   (Katie G.)

What I Ate: —————— **Monday** ——————

MORNING   AFTERNOON   EVENING

Exercise / Accomplishments:

What I Ate: —————— **Tuesday** ——————

MORNING   AFTERNOON   EVENING

Exercise / Accomplishments:

What I Ate: —————— **Wednesday** ——————

MORNING   AFTERNOON   EVENING

Exercise / Accomplishments:

What I Ate: —————— **Thursday** ——————

MORNING   AFTERNOON   EVENING

Exercise / Accomplishments:

What I Ate: ——————— Friday ———————

MORNING   AFTERNOON   EVENING

Exercise / Accomplishments:

What I Ate: ——————— Saturday ———————

MORNING   AFTERNOON   EVENING

Exercise / Accomplishments:

What I Ate: ——————— Sunday ———————

MORNING   AFTERNOON   EVENING

Exercise / Accomplishments:

——————— What Really Helped This Week: ———————

Drink more, drink less.

"I've learned that when I think I'm hungry, I'm often just thirsty."
—*Leslie S. (72 pounds, 4 years)*

O FTEN, WHEN YOU START A DIET, you're told to drink a lot of water. Does it really do any good? It seems to help the masters fill up: Two out of three indicated that they make a concerted effort to drink water to control their weight. Don Mauer says, "I drink gallons of bottled spring water. It tastes good, and it's refreshing."

Some masters say that cutting back on alcohol is another way they control the amount of food they eat. With 7 calories per gram, alcohol comes close to fat, with its 9 calories per gram. Some masters limit their juice consumption because they'd rather "eat their calories than drink them."

This week, tune in to your beverage consumption:

❖ Try to drink 8 glasses of water each day. Keep a glass on your desk or on the counter at all times. If desired, make your water special by adding a twist of lemon or lime or using bottled spring water or sparkling water.

❖ If you're a wine- or cocktail-at-night person, consider cutting back to one or two nights a week. Have some flavored sparkling water instead.

❖ Keep track of any calorie-containing beverages—like regular soda, juice and alcoholic drinks—that you consume. Look up the calories to determine if this is how you want to spend them:

_____

_____

_____

Goal(s) for this week: _____

_____

_____

Anticipated Obstacles   **Possible Solutions**

_____   _____

_____   _____

_____   _____

Exercise Plan

Monday: _____

Tuesday: _____

Wednesday: _____

Thursday: _____

Friday: _____

Saturday: _____

Sunday: _____

Try This for Lunch

❖ **Bagel Sandwich:** 2 ounces shaved, smoked turkey breast on
1 onion bagel with lettuce and 1 tablespoon nonfat mayonnaise
❖ 1 large nectarine ❖ 8 ounces skim milk.

Calories: 392   Fat: 3.5 grams   (Tom F.)

What I Ate: ——————— Monday ———————

MORNING   AFTERNOON   EVENING

Exercise / Accomplishments:

What I Ate: ——————— Tuesday ———————

MORNING   AFTERNOON   EVENING

Exercise / Accomplishments:

What I Ate: ——————— Wednesday ———————

MORNING   AFTERNOON   EVENING

Exercise / Accomplishments:

What I Ate: ——————— Thursday ———————

MORNING   AFTERNOON   EVENING

Exercise / Accomplishments:

What I Ate: ———————— Friday ————————

MORNING   AFTERNOON   EVENING

Exercise / Accomplishments:

What I Ate: ———————— Saturday ————————

MORNING   AFTERNOON   EVENING

Exercise / Accomplishments:

What I Ate: ———————— Sunday ————————

MORNING   AFTERNOON   EVENING

Exercise / Accomplishments:

———————— What Really Helped This Week: ————————

IV

Feeling Better About Yourself

Getting Beyond
Food and Weight

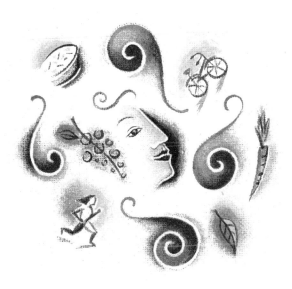

Learn to accept a less than perfect body.

"No matter how hard I work out, I will never have a body that looks muscular. But it's great to have a healthy cardiovascular system."

—*Ernie L. (40 pounds, 17 years)*

THE TRUTH IS that most people don't have perfect figures—even after they lose weight. But most masters manage to rejoice in their new bodies, despite any imperfections. For many, new clothing sizes and appearance are major motivations for staying thin.

To help yourself accept your body's shortcomings, **list several people you admire and/or find attractive who have "less than perfect" bodies, noting what it is that makes them attractive:**

_____

_____

_____

List one or more attractive aspects of your body, and take at least one step this week to enhance them. (For instance, if you have nice hands, paint your nails; if you have thick, shiny hair, get it restyled.)

_____

_____

_____

"By heritage, I have heavy calves. For years I tried to diminish their size only to finally find out that all I was doing was building more muscle. I get compliments on my size, so apparently my weight of 126 suits me."

—*Linda W. (44 pounds, 8 years)*

Goal(s) for this week: _____

_____

_____

Anticipated Obstacles	Possible Solutions
_____	_____
_____	_____
_____	_____

Exercise Plan

Monday: _____

Tuesday: _____

Wednesday: _____

Thursday: _____

Friday: _____

Saturday: _____

Sunday: _____

Try This for Supper

❖ **Joe's Simple Pasta and Vegetables:** Mix in a bowl 1 small sliced onion, ½ medium green pepper (sliced) and ⅓ cup each broccoli florets, sliced carrots, zucchini slices and sliced mushrooms with 1 cup cooked spaghetti, 2 tablespoons reduced-calorie Italian dressing, 2 tablespoons grated Parmesan cheese and garlic salt to taste; microwave. ❖ 1-ounce slice French bread with 1 teaspoon margarine.

Calories: 496   Fat: 13 grams   (Joe K.)

What I Ate: ———————— Monday ————————

MORNING · · · · · · · · · · · AFTERNOON · · · · · · · · · · · EVENING

Exercise / Accomplishments:

What I Ate: ———————— Tuesday ————————

MORNING · · · · · · · · · · · AFTERNOON · · · · · · · · · · · EVENING

Exercise / Accomplishments:

What I Ate: ———————— Wednesday ————————

MORNING · · · · · · · · · · · AFTERNOON · · · · · · · · · · · EVENING

Exercise / Accomplishments:

What I Ate: ———————— Thursday ————————

MORNING · · · · · · · · · · · AFTERNOON · · · · · · · · · · · EVENING

Exercise / Accomplishments:

Friday

What I Ate:

MORNING   AFTERNOON   EVENING

Exercise / Accomplishments:

Saturday

What I Ate:

MORNING   AFTERNOON   EVENING

Exercise / Accomplishments:

Sunday

What I Ate:

MORNING   AFTERNOON   EVENING

Exercise / Accomplishments:

What Really Helped This Week:

Realize that you are much more than your weight.

*"Life is not a beauty contest. Who cares if I weigh
130 or 140? I'm fine the way I am, and it isn't worth
giving up other things to focus on that."*

—*Vicki B. (56 pounds, 15 years)*

DO YOU OFTEN THINK THOUGHTS LIKE, "I'd be OK, if only
I could lose this weight?" It's time to realize that reaching your
goal weight isn't all there is to life.

Some studies suggest that having a good concept of self and a positive attitude are associated with losing and maintaining weight.
For some masters, like Vicki B., improved self-image came *before*
losing weight. She decided, "If I'm going to be this way, I'm going to
look nice. I started buying some nice 'fat' clothes for myself and
began to accept myself. Then the changes began."

How can you start to feel better about yourself right now?
**Make a list of things you like about yourself,
what you're good at and what others like or respect about you:**

_____

_____

_____

_____

*This week, each time you feel
discouraged, boost your self-esteem by
focusing on your positive attributes.*

Goal(s) for this week: _____

_____

_____

Anticipated Obstacles	Possible Solutions
_____	_____
_____	_____
_____	_____

Exercise Plan

Monday: _____

Tuesday: _____

Wednesday: _____

Thursday: _____

Friday: _____

Saturday: _____

Sunday: _____

Try This for a Snack

❖ **Large Iced Coffee:** 8 ounces skim milk, 1 cup strong coffee,
1 packet low-calorie sweetener (optional: add flavoring extracts,
such as vanilla, rum, amaretto, almond or mint).

Calories: 94   Fat: negligible   (Lynda M.)

What I Ate: ———————— **Monday** ————————

MORNING   AFTERNOON   EVENING

Exercise / Accomplishments:

What I Ate: ———————— **Tuesday** ————————

MORNING   AFTERNOON   EVENING

Exercise / Accomplishments:

What I Ate: ———————— **Wednesday** ————————

MORNING   AFTERNOON   EVENING

Exercise / Accomplishments:

What I Ate: ———————— **Thursday** ————————

MORNING   AFTERNOON   EVENING

Exercise / Accomplishments:

What I Ate: ——————— Friday ———————

MORNING   AFTERNOON   EVENING

Exercise / Accomplishments:

What I Ate: ——————— Saturday ———————

MORNING   AFTERNOON   EVENING

Exercise / Accomplishments:

What I Ate: ——————— Sunday ———————

MORNING   AFTERNOON   EVENING

Exercise / Accomplishments:

——————— What Really Helped This Week: ———————

Stop living for the day you'll be thin.

"When I first decided to do something about my weight, I was fundamentally dissatisfied with life. I was no longer happy as a field engineer, so I had a talk with 'the little boy' inside me. One of the things that I always wanted to be was a fireman. So I became one."

—*Tom F. (65 pounds, 20 years)*

Complete this sentence:
When I lose this weight, I'll . . .

_____

WHAT DO YOU FIND YOURSELF PUTTING OFF for the day you're finally "thin"? The problem with hinging life on your weight goal is that it gets in the way of feeling good about yourself.

Make a list of activities that you've thought about doing. Then rate their feasibility on a scale of 1 to 5, with 1 being "possible" and 5 being "impossible." Choose one that received a 1 or 2 and make a plan of action.

Activities I've thought about doing   Feasibility (1–5):

_____   _____

_____   _____

_____   _____

_____   _____

Plan of action:

_____

_____

_____

Weekly Forecast

Goal(s) for this week: _____

_____

_____

Anticipated Obstacles   **Possible Solutions**

_____   _____

_____   _____

_____   _____

Exercise Plan

Monday: _____

Tuesday: _____

Wednesday: _____

Thursday: _____

Friday: _____

Saturday: _____

Sunday: _____

Try This for Breakfast

❖ 2 slices cinnamon-raisin toast, each spread with 2 tablespoons
warm applesauce (unsweetened) and sprinkled with cinnamon

❖ 8 ounces skim milk.

Calories: 294   Fat: 4.5 grams   (Nancy K.)

What I Ate: ———————— Monday ————————

MORNING   AFTERNOON   EVENING

Exercise / Accomplishments:

What I Ate: ———————— Tuesday ————————

MORNING   AFTERNOON   EVENING

Exercise / Accomplishments:

What I Ate: ———————— Wednesday ————————

MORNING   AFTERNOON   EVENING

Exercise / Accomplishments:

What I Ate: ———————— Thursday ————————

MORNING   AFTERNOON   EVENING

Exercise / Accomplishments:

What I Ate: ———————— Friday ————————

MORNING   AFTERNOON   EVENING

Exercise / Accomplishments:

What I Ate: ———————— Saturday ————————

MORNING   AFTERNOON   EVENING

Exercise / Accomplishments:

What I Ate: ———————— Sunday ————————

MORNING   AFTERNOON   EVENING

Exercise / Accomplishments:

———————— What Really Helped This Week: ————————

Get more out of life.

"When I was gaining weight, I wouldn't go out because someone might see me. So I stayed home and ate and felt sorry for myself. Once I figured out what was happening, I decided to break out. Having fun and feeling good were more important!"

—***Tami B. (30 pounds, 8 years)***

HOW MUCH TIME DO YOU SPEND doing things you feel you *have* to do versus things you *want* to do? Many of the masters donned protective armor against weight regain by developing more fulfilled and interesting lives. *They found a way to get more out of life.*

So that your life revolves less around food and weight control, it's important to find new ways of enjoying yourself. Make a list of small things you enjoy but seldom take the time to do.

Bob W.'s list includes sharing a cup of tea with a friend, singing songs, looking at the stars, watching his garden grow and playing with his dog.

Make a special effort to do at least one pleasurable thing each day this week.

20 Small Pleasures:

_____

_____

_____

_____

_____

_____

Weekly Forecast

Goal(s) for this week: _____

_____

_____

Anticipated Obstacles	Possible Solutions
_____	_____
_____	_____
_____	_____

Exercise Plan

Monday: _____

Tuesday: _____

Wednesday: _____

Thursday: _____

Friday: _____

Saturday: _____

Sunday: _____

Try This for Lunch

❖ 8-inch whole wheat tortilla spread with 2 tablespoons fat-free "refried" beans and warmed. Top with 2 tablespoons chopped onion, ½ medium tomato (sliced), 2 tablespoons salsa, ¼ cup shredded reduced-fat cheddar cheese, 1 tablespoon nonfat sour cream. ❖ 3 slices fresh or canned juice-packed pineapple.

Calories: 391   Fat: 9 grams   (Bonnie R.)

What I Ate: ——————— Monday ———————

MORNING   AFTERNOON   EVENING

Exercise / Accomplishments:

What I Ate: ——————— Tuesday ———————

MORNING   AFTERNOON   EVENING

Exercise / Accomplishments:

What I Ate: ——————— Wednesday ———————

MORNING   AFTERNOON   EVENING

Exercise / Accomplishments:

What I Ate: ——————— Thursday ———————

MORNING   AFTERNOON   EVENING

Exercise / Accomplishments:

What I Ate: ——————— Friday ———————

MORNING   AFTERNOON   EVENING

Exercise / Accomplishments:

What I Ate: ——————— Saturday ———————

MORNING   AFTERNOON   EVENING

Exercise / Accomplishments:

What I Ate: ——————— Sunday ———————

MORNING   AFTERNOON   EVENING

Exercise / Accomplishments:

——————— What Really Helped This Week: ———————

Put yourself first, at least some of the time.

"When I was always trying to meet everyone else's needs, there was a big hole inside of me. I filled it up with food. Now I make an effort to know my own needs, wants and desires, in addition to helping others."

—*Jennifer P. (56 pounds, 15 years)*

JENNIFER BELIEVES that in order to lose weight permanently, she had to learn to put herself first. Like her, many masters said that in the past the only "nice" thing they did for themselves was to indulge in food.

She now treats herself with movies, clothes, activities with her kids and a monthly women's group. For each 10-pound loss, Don Mauer bought himself a compact disk or a tape.

List below at least five ways you can reward yourself without food:

_____

_____

_____

_____

_____

Each day this week, make three separate lists: 1. things you absolutely have to do; 2. things you want to do for yourself and 3. things that can wait.

Be sure to do at least one or two things for yourself each day.

"I may take a whole day and pamper myself, do whatever I want to do."

—*Irene S. (77 pounds, 5 years)*

Goal(s) for this week: _____

_____

_____

Anticipated Obstacles	Possible Solutions
_____	_____
_____	_____
_____	_____

Exercise Plan

Monday: _____

Tuesday: _____

Wednesday: _____

Thursday: _____

Friday: _____

Saturday: _____

Sunday: _____

Try This for Supper

❖ 4 ounces grilled or broiled skinless chicken breast with 2 tablespoons barbecue sauce ❖ 1 cup steamed green beans, seasoned with liquid smoke ❖ 1 cup corn ❖ 1 medium baked potato, flavored with Molly McButter, salt and pepper.

Calories: 500   Fat: 5 grams   (Teresa M.)

What I Ate: ——————— Monday ———————

MORNING   AFTERNOON   EVENING

Exercise / Accomplishments:

What I Ate: ——————— Tuesday ———————

MORNING   AFTERNOON   EVENING

Exercise / Accomplishments:

What I Ate: ——————— Wednesday ———————

MORNING   AFTERNOON   EVENING

Exercise / Accomplishments:

What I Ate: ——————— Thursday ———————

MORNING   AFTERNOON   EVENING

Exercise / Accomplishments:

What I Ate: — Friday —

MORNING   AFTERNOON   EVENING

Exercise / Accomplishments:

What I Ate: — Saturday —

MORNING   AFTERNOON   EVENING

Exercise / Accomplishments:

What I Ate: — Sunday —

MORNING   AFTERNOON   EVENING

Exercise / Accomplishments:

What Really Helped This Week:

Learn the art of positive self-talk.

*"In the past, if I gained a pound, it would ruin my day.
I'd feel that I'd failed and I would have to decrease my calories
even more. Now if I gain a little, I say to myself, 'I know I'm eating
the same amount and have the same amount of activity.' I realize
the gain is temporary, and I'm confident I'll go back down.*

—*Joanna M. (51 pounds, 12 years)*

MANY OF US ENGAGE IN NEGATIVE SELF-TALK—destructive thoughts—that trigger us to overeat. Self-talk is that conversation you constantly have with yourself. As Kelly S. puts it, "We all have tapes running through our heads." Negative self-talk can lead to inappropriate eating. The masters have learned to make their self-talk positive, which, in turn, helps them control their eating and their weight.

This week, each time you have the urge to eat in a way that's inconsistent with your goals, ask yourself what you're thinking.

If the self-talk is negative, turn it into a positive statement. For instance, tell yourself that you *can* do it, you're *not* going to gain the weight back, you're *not* a slob, it *won't* be the end of the world if you choose not to eat something and you're not the only one who has to watch what you eat.

**Record below some samples of *your* negative self-talk
and how you made it positive:**

_____

_____

_____

_____

_____

Weekly Forecast

Goal(s) for this week: _____

_____

_____

Anticipated Obstacles   **Possible Solutions**

_____   _____

_____   _____

_____   _____

Exercise Plan

Monday: _____

Tuesday: _____

Wednesday: _____

Thursday: _____

Friday: _____

Saturday: _____

Sunday: _____

Try This for Dessert

❖ 2-ounce piece angel food cake with ½ cup sliced fresh
strawberries and 2 tablespoons reduced-fat dessert topping.

        Calories: 191   Fat: 2 grams   (Ann F.)

What I Ate: ——————— Monday ———————

MORNING   AFTERNOON   EVENING

Exercise / Accomplishments:

What I Ate: ——————— Tuesday ———————

MORNING   AFTERNOON   EVENING

Exercise / Accomplishments:

What I Ate: ——————— Wednesday ———————

MORNING   AFTERNOON   EVENING

Exercise / Accomplishments:

What I Ate: ——————— Thursday ———————

MORNING   AFTERNOON   EVENING

Exercise / Accomplishments:

What I Ate: ———————— Friday ————————

MORNING   AFTERNOON   EVENING

Exercise / Accomplishments:

What I Ate: ———————— Saturday ————————

MORNING   AFTERNOON   EVENING

Exercise / Accomplishments:

What I Ate: ———————— Sunday ————————

MORNING   AFTERNOON   EVENING

Exercise / Accomplishments:

———————— What Really Helped This Week: ————————

Celebrate the present, but never forget the past.

*"I remind myself every day how far I've come by looking at myself
in the mirror or weighing myself. I remember what it was like when
I was heavy: that I couldn't even walk a block, much less do a step class
for one solid hour! I constantly think of how it used to be and
how I am now a happy, healthy and energetic person."*

—Peppi S. (27 pounds, 9 years)

I T'S QUITE EASY TO BE MOTIVATED when weight loss is new. Everyone notices, and you've got a whole new set of clothes. But with time, the compliments taper off; some people don't even know you were once heavy. *The masters stay motivated by recalling the pain of being heavy and never forgetting why they lost the weight.*

This is not the same as dwelling on past failures. It is recalling the pain of being heavy in an effort to keep from going back to your old habits.

In addition, the masters continually remind themselves of their accomplishments. "I recall the extraordinary moments when I found the clothes in the big men's shop were too big for me *and* when I could purchase health insurance at a normal rate. Thinking of this keeps me motivated," says Don Mauer.

Make a list of all the things you like better about yourself already, even if you're not at your goal weight. Be sure to note benefits such as having more energy, sleeping better, having more confidence, feeling less bloated and becoming more fit.

_____

_____

_____

Anytime you hit a plateau or feel discouraged, pull out your list.

Weekly Forecast

Goal(s) for this week: _____

_____

_____

Anticipated Obstacles   Possible Solutions

_____   _____

_____   _____

_____   _____

Exercise Plan

Monday: _____

Tuesday: _____

Wednesday: _____

Thursday: _____

Friday: _____

Saturday: _____

Sunday: _____

Try This for Breakfast

❖ 2 fat-free waffles, topped with 1 teaspoon real butter and

2 tablespoons reduced-calorie pancake syrup ❖ ½ grapefruit.

Calories: 296   Fat: 4 grams   (Cindy P.)

What I Ate: ——————— Monday ———————

MORNING   AFTERNOON   EVENING

Exercise / Accomplishments:

What I Ate: ——————— Tuesday ———————

MORNING   AFTERNOON   EVENING

Exercise / Accomplishments:

What I Ate: ——————— Wednesday ———————

MORNING   AFTERNOON   EVENING

Exercise / Accomplishments:

What I Ate: ——————— Thursday ———————

MORNING   AFTERNOON   EVENING

Exercise / Accomplishments:

What I Ate: —————————— Friday ——————————

MORNING   AFTERNOON   EVENING

Exercise / Accomplishments:

What I Ate: —————————— Saturday ——————————

MORNING   AFTERNOON   EVENING

Exercise / Accomplishments:

What I Ate: —————————— Sunday ——————————

MORNING   AFTERNOON   EVENING

Exercise / Accomplishments:

—————————— What Really Helped This Week: ——————————

V

Facing Life's Challenges

Coping with Problem Times, Problem People

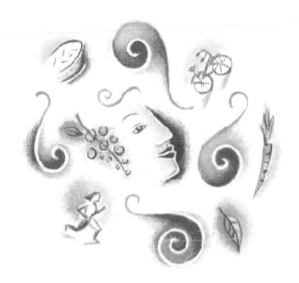

Cope with your tough time of day.

*"I try to occupy my evening with something
constructive that I enjoy—a good book, a good movie,
some computer work at home or going out with
friends to a noneating function."*

—*Jim V. (235 pounds, 5 years)*

I F YOU'RE LIKE MOST MASTERS, you have a tough time of day, when it's difficult to control your eating. Stop and think about when *your* tough time is. How can you learn to handle it better? The masters' most popular strategy is to do something other than eat. Here's their list of options:

Call a friend.

Go for a walk.

Get involved in a hobby.

Go to bed.

Take a hot bath.

Read a book or magazine.

Brush your teeth.

Stay out of the kitchen.

Get out of the house.

Make love.

Drink a no-cal beverage.

Other ways that the masters handle their tough times are to have low-fat foods or beverages. Some, like Kay D., save a treat for that time of day. Finally, when the urge to eat hits, some masters make an effort to sort out their feelings.

**This week, make a note on your food diary
of how you handled your tough time each day.**

Goal(s) for this week: _____

_____

_____

Anticipated Obstacles   **Possible Solutions**

_____   _____

_____   _____

_____   _____

Exercise Plan

Monday: _____

Tuesday: _____

Wednesday: _____

Thursday: _____

Friday: _____

Saturday: _____

Sunday: _____

Try This for Lunch

❖ **Hearty Club Sandwich:** 2 slices rye bread (toasted), 2 ounces sliced smoked turkey breast, 1 thin slice (½ ounce) Swiss cheese, ½ medium tomato (sliced), 3 green pepper slices, 1 romaine lettuce leaf, 4 cucumber slices, 1 tablespoon reduced-fat mayonnaise ❖ 1 watermelon wedge (1-x-5-inch slice).

Calories: 373   Fat: 10.5 grams   (Carol W.)

WEEK

43

What I Ate: ——————— **Monday** ———————

MORNING   AFTERNOON   EVENING

Exercise / Accomplishments:

What I Ate: ——————— **Tuesday** ———————

MORNING   AFTERNOON   EVENING

Exercise / Accomplishments:

What I Ate: ——————— **Wednesday** ———————

MORNING   AFTERNOON   EVENING

Exercise / Accomplishments:

What I Ate: ——————— **Thursday** ———————

MORNING   AFTERNOON   EVENING

Exercise / Accomplishments:

What I Ate: ———————— Friday ————————

MORNING   AFTERNOON   EVENING

Exercise / Accomplishments:

What I Ate: ———————— Saturday ————————

MORNING   AFTERNOON   EVENING

Exercise / Accomplishments:

What I Ate: ———————— Sunday ————————

MORNING   AFTERNOON   EVENING

Exercise / Accomplishments:

———————— What Really Helped This Week: ————————

Handle your emotions and problems without food.

*"I recognize my hungers for what they are.
When my stomach growls, I eat. When I'm feeling down or sad,
I call a friend or read a book or hop on my rollerblades—or drink
a beer, cry a little and go to sleep! When my soul feels empty, I pick
up a pen and write out what's going on inside of me."*

—Katie G. (30 pounds, 7 years)

THE MASTERS HAVE LEARNED to deal with emotions and problems other than by eating. Bob W. asks himself, "What do I really need right now? To talk with someone? To rest? A hug? A pleasant activity? A cup of tea shared with a friend?" If you're angry, it may help to get some exercise or deal directly with your anger. If you're bored or lonely, try getting out of the house. Call a supportive friend, go for a walk or go tinker in your garden for a few hours.

**This week, each time you have the desire to eat for a reason
other than hunger, follow this three-step process:**

1. Label your feelings or identify your problem.
2. Ask yourself if eating will really solve your problem.
3. Get involved in an alternate activity—something that will truly make you feel better.

Date	Emotion or problem	Alternate activity

Goal(s) for this week: _____

_____

_____

Anticipated Obstacles   **Possible Solutions**

_____   _____

_____   _____

_____   _____

Exercise Plan

Monday: _____

Tuesday: _____

Wednesday: _____

Thursday: _____

Friday: _____

Saturday: _____

Sunday: _____

Try This for Supper

❖ **4 baked chicken nuggets:** 3-ounce boneless chicken breast, cut into 4 pieces and dipped in ¼ cup buttermilk, then in ¼ cup seasoned bread crumbs ❖ ¾ cup cooked angel hair pasta with 1 tablespoon pesto and 2 tablespoons sun-dried tomatoes ❖ ½ cup Italian green beans, steamed ❖ 1 slice watermelon (1-x-5-inch slice).

Calories: 493   **Fat: 11 grams**   (Connye Z.)

What I Ate: ———————— Monday ————————————

MORNING   AFTERNOON   EVENING

Exercise / Accomplishments:

What I Ate: ———————— Tuesday ————————————

MORNING   AFTERNOON   EVENING

Exercise / Accomplishments:

What I Ate: ———————— Wednesday ————————

MORNING   AFTERNOON   EVENING

Exercise / Accomplishments:

What I Ate: ———————— Thursday ————————————

MORNING   AFTERNOON   EVENING

Exercise / Accomplishments:

What I Ate: ———————— Friday ————————

MORNING   AFTERNOON   EVENING

Exercise / Accomplishments:

What I Ate: ———————— Saturday ————————

MORNING   AFTERNOON   EVENING

Exercise / Accomplishments:

What I Ate: ———————— Sunday ————————

MORNING   AFTERNOON   EVENING

Exercise / Accomplishments:

———————— What Really Helped This Week: ————————

Cut your losses.

"I've learned to forgive myself when I blow my eating plan and get back on track as soon as I can. The 'old' me would have used that as an excuse to keep on eating."

—Lynda M. (36 pounds, 13 years)

IT MAY COME AS A RELIEF TO KNOW that the masters are not perfect: they are *not* always 100 percent in control of tempting foods and how they handle life's difficult moments. But they don't punish themselves when they slip back into old ways and they don't allow occasional lapses to become a trigger for weight gain. When they don't handle a situation the way they would have liked, they forgive themselves and move on.

Ask yourself the following questions when you have a slip:

❖ What went wrong?
❖ How can I handle things differently next time?
❖ What can I do constructively to make up for the slip—without punishing myself?

Sometimes the best course of action is to forget about it and get right back on track.

*"I don't feel guilty if I overeat one day.
If you let yourself feel guilty, you just eat more."*

—Jean B. (53 pounds, 9 years)

Weekly Forecast

Goal(s) for this week: _____

_____

_____

Anticipated Obstacles   **Possible Solutions**

_____   _____

_____   _____

_____   _____

Exercise Plan

Monday: _____

Tuesday: _____

Wednesday: _____

Thursday: _____

Friday: _____

Saturday: _____

Sunday: _____

Try This for Breakfast

❖ ½ cup nonfat cottage cheese on a bed of fruit: ½ peach, 10 red grapes, ½ medium pear, ½ cup sliced strawberries ❖ 1 slice whole wheat cinnamon-raisin toast with 1 teaspoon nonfat margarine.

Calories: 295   Fat: 2.5 grams   (Bob W.)

What I Ate: ——————— Monday ———————

MORNING　　　　AFTERNOON　　　　EVENING

Exercise / Accomplishments:

What I Ate: ——————— Tuesday ———————

MORNING　　　　AFTERNOON　　　　EVENING

Exercise / Accomplishments:

What I Ate: ——————— Wednesday ———————

MORNING　　　　AFTERNOON　　　　EVENING

Exercise / Accomplishments:

What I Ate: ——————— Thursday ———————

MORNING　　　　AFTERNOON　　　　EVENING

Exercise / Accomplishments:

What I Ate: ——————— Friday ———————

MORNING AFTERNOON EVENING

Exercise / Accomplishments:

What I Ate: ——————— Saturday ———————

MORNING AFTERNOON EVENING

Exercise / Accomplishments:

What I Ate: ——————— Sunday ———————

MORNING AFTERNOON EVENING

Exercise / Accomplishments:

——————— What Really Helped This Week: ———————

Nip small weight gains in the bud.

"I normally weigh myself once or twice a week.
But if I feel like my weight is up, judging by the fit of my clothes,
I won't weigh for a few days to see if I can make some adjustments.
I exercise more, reduce portions and pay more attention to fat content.
I know if I spend several days watching it, I'll be back down."

—*Janice C. (43 pounds, 18 years)*

AT LAST! You're finally at your goal. But you find yourself loosening up, and before you know it, you've gained back 5 pounds. The masters monitor their weight, usually by regular weigh-ins, and if they gain just a small amount, they *immediately* take it off. The vast majority stop gaining before they put on more than 5 pounds; most others allow themselves no more than 10. If they do gain a little weight back, nearly every master has a game plan for getting back down.

If you're going to keep small gains from getting out of hand, you need some means of monitoring your weight. Next, you need to establish your own weight "buffer zone," a range in which you feel comfortable—but no more than 5 to 10 pounds above your goal. Finally, have a game plan for getting your weight back down (step up exercise, decrease sweets, keep a diary, reduce portions).

Remind yourself that it's a lot less painful to deal with 5 or 10
pounds at a time than it is 30, 50 or 100 pounds.

Buffer Zone: _____

Game Plan for Losing: _____

_____

_____

Goal(s) for this week: _____

_____

_____

Anticipated Obstacles	Possible Solutions
_____	_____
_____	_____
_____	_____

Exercise Plan

Monday: _____

Tuesday: _____

Wednesday: _____

Thursday: _____

Friday: _____

Saturday: _____

Sunday: _____

Try This for Lunch

❖ **Pasta Salad:** Mix ¾ cup cooked rotini pasta, ¼ cup sliced
fresh mushrooms and ½ cup mixed vegetables (steamed) with
2 tablespoons fat-free Italian dressing ❖ 1-ounce breadstick
❖ 2 apricots ❖ 8 ounces skim milk.

Calories: 374   Fat: 3 grams   (Debbie T.)

What I Ate: ——————— Monday ———————

MORNING   AFTERNOON   EVENING

Exercise / Accomplishments:

What I Ate: ——————— Tuesday ———————

MORNING   AFTERNOON   EVENING

Exercise / Accomplishments:

What I Ate: ——————— Wednesday ———————

MORNING   AFTERNOON   EVENING

Exercise / Accomplishments:

What I Ate: ——————— Thursday ———————

MORNING   AFTERNOON   EVENING

Exercise / Accomplishments:

Friday

What I Ate:

MORNING   AFTERNOON   EVENING

Exercise / Accomplishments:

Saturday

What I Ate:

MORNING   AFTERNOON   EVENING

Exercise / Accomplishments:

Sunday

What I Ate:

MORNING   AFTERNOON   EVENING

Exercise / Accomplishments:

What Really Helped This Week:

Learn to say no.

*"When people push food on me, I politely say,
'Thanks, but no thanks. I don't want to carry
that old body around again.'"*

—*Chuck B. (60 pounds, 8 years)*

WHAT DO YOU DO WHEN SOMEONE PUSHES FOOD ON YOU?
Nancy G. admits, "It takes time to get past the comments,
'You're thin enough,' 'A little dessert won't hurt you,' 'How can
you eat that many vegetables?' or 'It would be so much easier if
you ate what everyone else does.'" She is describing all-too-famil-
iar comments from individuals who, knowingly or unknowingly, attempt to sabotage slimmed-down people.

When I asked the masters how they go about handling food
pushers, most of them said they politely decline the offer. Some masters find it helps to make others aware of their weight-loss success.
Others may take a small amount. When polite refusals don't work,
the masters just become more direct. Rosemary O. tells her mother,
"If you ask me again, I'll just have to keep saying 'no.'" *The masters make it clear that they don't let food pushers push them around.*

When all else fails, blame it on your health or use humor. Virginia
L. baffles people with her line, "I have chronic food intolerance,"
while Katie G. quips, "If I eat any more, I'll throw up all over your
new Nike running shoes."

Record your one-liners for turning away food pushers:

_____

_____

_____

Weekly Forecast

Goal(s) for this week: _____

_____

_____

Anticipated Obstacles   Possible Solutions

_____   _____

_____   _____

_____   _____

Exercise Plan

Monday: _____

Tuesday: _____

Wednesday: _____

Thursday: _____

Friday: _____

Saturday: _____

Sunday: _____

Try This for Supper

❖ **Linguine with Shrimp and Vegetables:** Toss together 1 cup cooked linguine, 3 ounces steamed shrimp, ⅓ cup each steamed broccoli florets, mushrooms and carrot coins and 1 large clove garlic, minced and sautéed in 1 teaspoon olive oil. Sprinkle with basil and 1 tablespoon grated Parmesan cheese. ❖ 1½ cups romaine lettuce with ¼ cup sliced water chestnuts and 2 tablespoons reduced-fat creamy Italian dressing.

Calories: 490   Fat: 13 grams   (Lynda M.)

What I Ate: —————————— Monday ——————————

MORNING   AFTERNOON   EVENING

Exercise / Accomplishments:

What I Ate: —————————— Tuesday ——————————

MORNING   AFTERNOON   EVENING

Exercise / Accomplishments:

What I Ate: —————————— Wednesday ——————————

MORNING   AFTERNOON   EVENING

Exercise / Accomplishments:

What I Ate: —————————— Thursday ——————————

MORNING   AFTERNOON   EVENING

Exercise / Accomplishments:

What I Ate: —————————— Friday ——————————

MORNING   AFTERNOON   EVENING

Exercise / Accomplishments:

What I Ate: —————————— Saturday ——————————

MORNING   AFTERNOON   EVENING

Exercise / Accomplishments:

What I Ate: —————————— Sunday ——————————

MORNING   AFTERNOON   EVENING

Exercise / Accomplishments:

————————— What Really Helped This Week: —————————

Cope with family members who eat differently.

*"My husband can eat anything he wants—
usually it's something fat, sweet, creamy. But I have
my own side of the fridge with my allowable kinds of food.
Sometimes he likes my 'goodies' better!"*

—*Virginia L. (97 pounds, 4 years)*

WHAT DO YOU DO WHEN YOU EAT NO FAT, but they eat no lean? Some masters live with overweight people who make no effort to change their eating habits, while others have family members who don't really need to watch their weight.

**This week, think about which of the following masters'
strategies would work best in your home:**

❖ *Eat less of what they eat.* Quite a few masters eat what their families eat, but in smaller quantities. They then fill up on low-calorie side dishes. Joy C. says, "I add a big tossed salad or cabbage salad, plus a vegetable and a starch like potatoes or rice."

❖ *Eat something different.* Some masters eat different food from their families or spouses, at least some of the time. They may cook low-fat versions of what they're serving others for themselves.

❖ *Avoid certain of their foods.* Some masters view certain foods as "theirs, not mine." Joanna M. makes this easier by trying to buy food for her children that she's not wild about.

❖ *Win them over to healthful eating by preparing tasty low-fat recipes or by making favorite dishes lower in fat.* Eileen K. declares, "I told my family this is the way I cook now. If they want something else, they can make it on their own."

Goal(s) for this week: _____

_____

_____

Anticipated Obstacles   **Possible Solutions**

_____   _____

_____   _____

_____   _____

Exercise Plan

Monday: _____

Tuesday: _____

Wednesday: _____

Thursday: _____

Friday: _____

Saturday: _____

Sunday: _____

Try This for a Snack

❖ 6 reduced-fat cinnamon crisp graham cracker squares with

2 tablespoons nonfat cream cheese.

Calories: 195   Fat: 2.5 grams   (Emil R.)

Monday

What I Ate:

MORNING   AFTERNOON   EVENING

Exercise / Accomplishments:

Tuesday

What I Ate:

MORNING   AFTERNOON   EVENING

Exercise / Accomplishments:

Wednesday

What I Ate:

MORNING   AFTERNOON   EVENING

Exercise / Accomplishments:

Thursday

What I Ate:

MORNING   AFTERNOON   EVENING

Exercise / Accomplishments:

Friday

What I Ate:

MORNING   AFTERNOON   EVENING

Exercise / Accomplishments:

Saturday

What I Ate:

MORNING   AFTERNOON   EVENING

Exercise / Accomplishments:

Sunday

What I Ate:

MORNING   AFTERNOON   EVENING

Exercise / Accomplishments:

What Really Helped This Week:

Find new things to do with former food buddies.

"Some of my friends look up to me as an example of success, others point me out as a future failure, while still others accuse me of 'cheating' when I eat certain foods."

—*Stan J. (103 pounds, 5 years)*

As Stan's experience so aptly illustrates, it's not all praise and glory from friends when you lose weight. It may be especially hard to deal with old food buddies who are either jealous of you or who cannot accept your new habits. In their defense, when a relationship is focused on eating, it's tough to accept it when one party decides to change. But you don't have to end these food-based friendships.

Make a list of friends with whom you have a food relationship:

_____

_____

_____

The next time you get together with any of them, try one or more of the following masters' suggestions:

❖ Plan nonfood-related activities. Dorothy J. says, "We attend a play rather than eat together."

❖ "Recruit" them to exercise with you, as does Suzanne T., who adds, "You can encourage one another."

❖ Be assertive. Lolly D. explains, "Some of my friends still need to be reminded at times that I have to stick to these healthier changes even if they choose unhealthy foods."

Goal(s) for this week: _____

_____

_____

Anticipated Obstacles · · · · · Possible Solutions

_____ · · · · · _____

_____ · · · · · _____

_____ · · · · · _____

Exercise Plan

Monday: _____

Tuesday: _____

Wednesday: _____

Thursday: _____

Friday: _____

Saturday: _____

Sunday: _____

Try This for Breakfast

❖ 1 toasted oat-bran waffle, topped with ⅓ cup nonfat cottage cheese. Drizzle with 2 teaspoons honey and sprinkle with nutmeg

❖ 6 ounces orange juice.

Calories: 290 **Fat: 4 grams** (Ann Q.)

What I Ate: ——————— Monday ———————

MORNING   AFTERNOON   EVENING

Exercise / Accomplishments:

What I Ate: ——————— Tuesday ———————

MORNING   AFTERNOON   EVENING

Exercise / Accomplishments:

What I Ate: ——————— Wednesday ———————

MORNING   AFTERNOON   EVENING

Exercise / Accomplishments:

What I Ate: ——————— Thursday ———————

MORNING   AFTERNOON   EVENING

Exercise / Accomplishments:

What I Ate: ——————— Friday ———————

MORNING   AFTERNOON   EVENING

Exercise / Accomplishments:

What I Ate: ——————— Saturday ———————

MORNING   AFTERNOON   EVENING

Exercise / Accomplishments:

What I Ate: ——————— Sunday ———————

MORNING   AFTERNOON   EVENING

Exercise / Accomplishments:

——————— What Really Helped This Week: ———————

Plan ahead for special occasions.

"I avoid restaurants where there are no good choices.
It's too hard for me to eat a little bit. Now, if someone asks me
where I'd like to go, I never say, 'Wherever you want.'
I choose because I don't want to be set up to overeat."

—*Joanne F. (80 pounds, 8 years)*

THE MASTERS HAVE MANY CREATIVE WAYS OF COPING with special occasions. When it comes to restaurants, seven out of ten masters dine out at least once or twice a week. Most, however, avoid all-you-can-eat buffets and fast food restaurants. They don't hesitate to make special requests as well as inquire about how foods are prepared. They often bring along their own low-fat condiments, like salad dressing.

At social occasions like dinners, parties and weddings, the masters have a small amount of what's offered but focus on socializing rather than on eating. Quite a few are selective. JoAnna L. says, "I look at everything before putting anything on my plate. I make the best decisions based on what there is, and I don't go back for seconds."

When the masters go on vacation, many make an effort to do the same things they do at home to control their weight. Ann F. says, "I like to snack and visit candy stores, so I try to have fruit for breakfast."

Try to anticipate: Have at least a rough game plan anytime you're going to a restaurant, party or on vacation. If you splurge, don't feel guilty; make a trade-off by compensating at another meal or getting some extra exercise.

"When I'm on vacation, I try to remember that
I'll be returning with the same old body. There's no free lunch."

—*Tim H. (25 pounds, 10 years)*

Weekly Forecast

Goal(s) for this week: _____

_____

_____

Anticipated Obstacles   **Possible Solutions**

_____   _____

_____   _____

_____   _____

Exercise Plan

Monday: _____

Tuesday: _____

Wednesday: _____

Thursday: _____

Friday: _____

Saturday: _____

Sunday: _____

Try This for Supper

❖ 4 ounces steamed salmon ❖ 1 cup asparagus ❖ 1 medium baked
potato (4 ounces) with 1 pat butter ❖ **Spinach Salad:** 2 cups fresh
spinach, 2 slices red onion, ⅓ cup sliced fresh mushrooms,
1 teaspoon bacon bits, 1 tablespoon honey-Dijon dressing.

Calories: 499   Fat: 17 grams   (Leslie S.)

What I Ate: ———————— ## Monday ————————

MORNING   AFTERNOON   EVENING

Exercise / Accomplishments:

What I Ate: ———————— ## Tuesday ————————

MORNING   AFTERNOON   EVENING

Exercise / Accomplishments:

What I Ate: ———————— ## Wednesday ————————

MORNING   AFTERNOON   EVENING

Exercise / Accomplishments:

What I Ate: ———————— ## Thursday ————————

MORNING   AFTERNOON   EVENING

Exercise / Accomplishments:

What I Ate: ——————— Friday ———————

MORNING   AFTERNOON   EVENING

Exercise / Accomplishments:

What I Ate: ——————— Saturday ———————

MORNING   AFTERNOON   EVENING

Exercise / Accomplishments:

What I Ate: ——————— Sunday ———————

MORNING   AFTERNOON   EVENING

Exercise / Accomplishments:

——————— What Really Helped This Week: ———————

Look for the warning signs.

*"In the past, I'd use any excuse to 'blow it all off.' Now, if I gain
5 pounds, my maintenance group helps head me off. Sometimes
it's useful to hear someone say, 'Why don't you try this again?'
The broader your repertoire of tricks, the better you are
at keeping weight off."*

—*Jim J. (165 pounds, 7 years)*

MAINTENANCE IS NOT just a matter of reaching a number on
a scale, then staying there. Maintenance includes staying with
all of the factors that brought you success in the first place—like
sticking with your exercise goals, continuing to manage problems
in new ways, developing new pleasures in life and not going back
to your old ways with food. It's about accepting that you have to
keep doing these things for the rest of your life.

But maintenance can be frustrating and trying at times, and you
may find yourself slipping and feeling less in control of your weight.

Look for the following warning signs that
you may need support:

❖ You're 5 to 10 pounds over your goal weight and cannot seem
to lose them.

❖ Your "thin" clothes are getting tight, and you find yourself
buying new, bigger clothes.

❖ Your old "tricks" that used to help are no longer effective.

❖ You find yourself turning to food to handle stress.

❖ Your mental attitude has changed, and you get lazy.

❖ You feel hopeless about your weight or out of control.

If the warning signs "fit," it's time to go back to the group or person who helped you lose weight, to find a weight-control buddy or
to confide in a relative or spouse who encourages you.

Goal(s) for this week: _____

_____

_____

Anticipated Obstacles   **Possible Solutions**

_____   _____

_____   _____

_____   _____

Exercise Plan

Monday: _____

Tuesday: _____

Wednesday: _____

Thursday: _____

Friday: _____

Saturday: _____

Sunday: _____

Try This for Dessert

❖ **Baked Apple:** Microwave 1 medium apple stuffed with 2
tablespoons raisins and sprinkled with cinnamon. Serve with 3
tablespoons fat-free vanilla yogurt.

Calories: 188   **Fat: negligible**   **(Edith S.)**

What I Ate: ———————— Monday ————————

MORNING   AFTERNOON   EVENING

Exercise / Accomplishments:

What I Ate: ———————— Tuesday ————————

MORNING   AFTERNOON   EVENING

Exercise / Accomplishments:

What I Ate: ———————— Wednesday ————————

MORNING   AFTERNOON   EVENING

Exercise / Accomplishments:

What I Ate: ———————— Thursday ————————

MORNING   AFTERNOON   EVENING

Exercise / Accomplishments:

What I Ate: ——————— Friday ———————

MORNING   AFTERNOON   EVENING

Exercise / Accomplishments:

What I Ate: ——————— Saturday ———————

MORNING   AFTERNOON   EVENING

Exercise / Accomplishments:

What I Ate: ——————— Sunday ———————

MORNING   AFTERNOON   EVENING

Exercise / Accomplishments:

——————— What Really Helped This Week: ———————

Look at the big picture.

*"If I don't handle a situation as I would have liked,
I put it in perspective: One candy bar won't make me 20
pounds overweight. I look at the big picture. I remind myself
that there are a multitude of things I do—like eating breakfast,
exercising and drinking water—that help me maintain my weight.
That candy bar is a drop in the bucket."*

—*Janice C. (43 pounds, 18 years)*

WHEN YOUR SUCCESS AT WEIGHT CONTROL is the result of meeting many small, achievable goals, it becomes more difficult to label any single "slip" as a failure. One mistake can't undo all your positive changes.

So set your sights on the small daily goals and achievements that lead to positive lifestyle change, such as healthful eating, more physical activity and feeling better about yourself.

**This week, take a moment each day to
reflect on the multiple small changes you've made
in your eating and exercise habits that ultimately
lead to long-term weight control:**

_____

_____

_____

_____

*"I give myself credit for my gains and try not to berate
myself. Instead of saying, 'I'm doing it wrong,' I say,
'I'm doing it more right than before.'"*

—*Tim H. (25 pounds, 10 years)*

Goal(s) for this week: _____

_____

_____

Anticipated Obstacles	Possible Solutions
_____	_____
_____	_____
_____	_____

Exercise Plan

Monday: _____

Tuesday: _____

Wednesday: _____

Thursday: _____

Friday: _____

Saturday: _____

Sunday: _____

Try This for Supper

❖ **Veggie Pizza:** 10-inch pita bread, spread with ⅓ cup reduced-fat spaghetti or pizza sauce, topped with ¼ cup each onions, green peppers, broccoli, zucchini and mushrooms that have been stir-fried in a nonstick skillet. Sprinkle with 1 tablespoon grated Parmesan cheese.

Calories: 489   Fat: 4 grams   (Chuck B.)

Monday

What I Ate:

MORNING   AFTERNOON   EVENING

Exercise / Accomplishments:

Tuesday

What I Ate:

MORNING   AFTERNOON   EVENING

Exercise / Accomplishments:

Wednesday

What I Ate:

MORNING   AFTERNOON   EVENING

Exercise / Accomplishments:

Thursday

What I Ate:

MORNING   AFTERNOON   EVENING

Exercise / Accomplishments:

What I Ate: —————— Friday ——————

MORNING   AFTERNOON   EVENING

Exercise / Accomplishments:

What I Ate: —————— Saturday ——————

MORNING   AFTERNOON   EVENING

Exercise / Accomplishments:

What I Ate: —————— Sunday ——————

MORNING   AFTERNOON   EVENING

Exercise / Accomplishments:

—————— What Really Helped This Week: ——————